DADSPIRATIONS:
THE 1ST

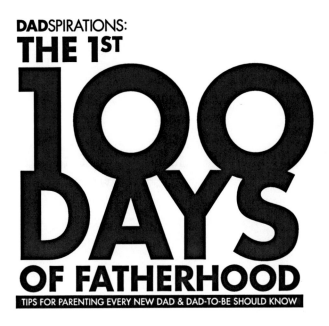

OF FATHERHOOD
TIPS FOR PARENTING EVERY NEW DAD & DAD-TO-BE SHOULD KNOW

by Pete Densmore

DADspirations:

THE FIRST 100 DAYS OF FATHERHOOD

ISBN: 978-0-615-66363-0

Cover design by Terry Lawrence
Editing, page design by Karen McChrystal
Photos by Pete Densmore

DADspirations Press
Bartlett, Illinois

Printed in the United States of America

CONTENTS

DADSPIRATIONS

Dedication

For my sweet loves—Bunsy, Cheeky and Munch.

Acknowledgments

Any wife who's okay with her husband spending every Tuesday night writing for six months moves into first place for Wife of the Year—thank you honey. To my two little ones, who inspire me every day, I can't wait for you to read this book and smile, or cringe. Ro-D and Tor, thank you for your lifetime of support; my thoughtfulness comes directly from you. To "E & A" for setting a great example with their amazing daughters, my nieces—and a special nod to Happy Amy for her amazing wit and humor. To the fathers of Stunt Dad and our Tuesday nights, thank you for helping me find my voice and crushing it every week. To Uncle Terry, you've made this book come alive. It would just be a bunch of words on paper without you. To Karen, my editor and helping hand throughout this entire process, I can't thank you enough for your patience, advice, and support along the way. And a special thank you to Mr. Gray for making sure my t's were crossed, i's were dotted, and for adding some much needed color commentary.

INTRODUCTION

Super Dad or Super Dud, it only takes 100 days to determine your fate...

Let's face it. As a new dad, you probably have no idea of what awaits you in the first few months of fatherhood, even if it's your second time around, because each kid is different and each experience is different. Regardless, you're a cool dude and you want to be that fun dad, yet you still might not want to believe that fun no longer means a brewskie and a ball game at noon. Since you're probably still figuring out how to put that crib together, this book is for you. I've been in the trenches, and to help my fellow man, I've come up with a strategy for the first 100 days that will rescue you from falling into the Super Dud trap and will show you how to be that Super Dad you really aspire to be.

This book is for the new father or father-to-be who wants a sneak peek into the months that lie ahead and wants to do some fun stuff for his little one, but either doesn't have the time to think about it or the time read about it. Like most dads, I prefer pictures and small words, so this has intentionally been written as a quick, conversational read for the guys, showing them how to impress their wives and shower their new arrival with the sweetest of fatherly gifts. When your wife starts bragging to her friends about the latest and greatest thing you did for baby, guess who's that much closer to getting a little nookie again?

On a more serious note, this book is also for the new mother or the mother-to-be who needs to, or is anticipating she will need to, give her spouse a swift kick in the behind in the proactive parenting department.

What you do in the first 100 days of being a father will give you a measure of how effective you're likely to be going forward. Your fathering efforts during this period will show you as well as your wife, family, and friends whether you're going to be a Super Dad or a Super Dud.

Fathers are most engaged when they experience the adrenaline rush of first becoming a new dad. Because everything is so new, the opportunity to shape your entire family is at its peak, and you have a strong desire to do everything you can for mom and baby. This desire has to do, in large part, with the fact that you haven't screwed up anything—yet. But you will my friend, and if you aren't heavily involved in fathering by the time you make the first of many inevitable mistakes, you're going to get frustrated and want to check out, which makes those first 100 days of fatherhood that much more critical.

The first 100 days is a common benchmark used to assess success and involvement, typically associated with U.S. presidents when they first take office. Although there might be days when you feel like you're facing the Great Diaper Depression or the Great Sleep Famine, you shouldn't feel that you are faced with a problem (i.e., baby). No, you are faced with the need for action, immediate action, like some of our nation's past leaders. And you have at least two people—mommy and baby—who need the reassurance that you are going to step up as man. In this particular situation, it's actually not about how you finish, it's how you start. Hey, it worked for Franklin D. Roosevelt (FDR) when he fathered a kind of rebirth of our country, pulling the U.S. out of the Great Depression with his 100-day New Deal program. If a 100-day program worked for reforming a country, why can't one work for fathering a newborn?

When preparing for the birth of my daughter, let's call her Marie, I was determined to have the same fatherly effectiveness as I had for my 18-month-old son. We'll call him Henry. Only after thinking about it in hindsight, I questioned how effective I truly was for him. Sure, I did my share of the diaper changing, the baby swaddling, and the middle of the night soothing, but was that enough to catapult me to Super Dad status? Did I put up a framed picture of him that first week back at work? Did I write down the first time he smiled? Did I set up a college fund for him?

A year and a half goes by as fast as a Nolan Ryan fastball, but nothing goes by faster than those first 100 days. And with my baby girl, I made it a point to do those things which I didn't know to do for my son. As the President of my household (or Vice President, should you ask my wife), I pledged a "New Deal" for my daughter. FDR is the only American president elected to more than two terms and is often regarded as one of the top U.S. Presidents, so who better to emulate? In keeping with FDR's legacy, I spearheaded weekly initiatives designed to *regard, remember* and *relish* this never-to-be-experienced-again time period. These "3 Rs" will benefit your wife and your baby. And through these activities, which I'll refer to as *DADspirations™*, you can bring many happy days to your own family.

I will break this 100-day stretch into two phases: the first thirteen weeks and then the Nine Days of Doting. For the first thirteen weeks of my daughter's life (days 1-91), I did two DADspirations each week: one for me (or my wife) and one for my daughter. If you have a son, you're in luck, because I've also identified how you can apply the DADspiration for my little girl for your little boy. But yes, it's true, I actually put myself first. However, that's not because I'm selfish. It was a way for me to keep my own sanity without going stark raving mad. And, no, weekly DADspirations for my daughter weren't my way of spoiling her; they were an outlet for me to express how much I care for her. And, for the final stretch (days 92-100), that week wasn't about me at all— just her. Nine adorably cute and insanely sweet things I did, just for her. Well, there might actually have been one thing I did for me that final week, but you'll have to keep reading to find out what that was.

This parenting book isn't meant to be intimidating or condescending. I'm not here to talk down to you. I, too, was once where you are at this moment: overwhelmed, excited, confused and already sick of people giving their two cents on which diaper holds the most crap. This is a book that is meant to inspire rather than instruct and to encourage rather than dictate. After all, you're a grown man, a husband, and either a new or a soon-to-be father. You don't need someone else telling you what to do.

MONTH 1

WEEK 1: REMEMBER IT WHILE YOU CAN

Time Capsule; Daddy Letter

You've read the *What To Expect When Expecting* book. You've graduated from the "Terrified of Having a Baby" class. You've practiced diapering everything from watermelons to the house cat. The nursery is painted with the colors your wife selected. The crib is built based on the instructions your wife gave you. And the rocker is positioned where your wife insisted. Congratulations, the hard part is over—you are officially ready for parenthood.

And fear not, this is one job that doesn't require experience, references or even a license.

When the big day finally arrives, you welcome your beautiful, amazing, adorable baby into the world. You can't stop smiling, laughing and crying, and pretty soon, everything will become a blur, a distant memory. This was an event you insist was the best day of your life, yet even a few short weeks later, you will have difficulty remembering the exact details. Who delivered my baby? How long was my wife in labor? Did I cut the umbilical cord? How could the greatest day of my life become a fuzzy memory so quickly?

For starters, your initial visitors are going to be complete strangers. They are the mandatory hospital staff, or known to some as the New Arrival Nine. They introduce themselves something like this:

1. I'm the floor nurse. I'll show you how to swaddle your baby like a burrito.

2. I'm the nurse manager. I'll teach you how to keep your kid alive.

3. I'm the gynecologist. I'll take care of all the bleeding that you had no idea was a part of normal childbirth. Smelling salts, anyone?

4. I'm the hospital's pediatrician. I'll double check to see that your baby is still breathing, charging you a mere $600 for a six-minute visit. Congratulations!

5. I'm the hospital's lawyer. I'll gauge your intent on suing us.

6. I'm the anesthesiologist. I'll confirm that mom has the feeling back in her legs.

7. I'm the pediatrician. I'll schedule my new patient's first doctor visit.

8. I'm the hospital's records administrator. I'll verify whether you really do want to go forward with that name for your baby.

9. I'm the hospital photographer. I'll make you feel guilty for not spending $500 to capture your baby's closed eyes, until you cave to our offer.

If you make it through this stage and are still patting yourself on the pack for not passing out during the delivery (and if you did pass out, at least you didn't piss your pants, right?), kudos are in order. The kudos should fortify you for what comes next: the barrage of stuffed animals and mylar balloons, the arrival of family and friends. Even if you and your wife are only children or you haven't had a friend since high school, the number of visitors will be too many. We had just one set of parents, an aunt, an uncle, a random neighbor, a now ex-boss, and that was enough to make us want to pull our hair out. For the three days we were in the hospital, I recollect maybe a minute of it, because for the 60 seconds I actually got to hold my baby boy my mind wasn't on enjoying the moment; it was concentrating on the most important rule of being a new parent, more important than anything: don't drop the baby.

So, the Week 1 message is remember it while you can. Here are DADspirations to consider doing to help you preserve the precious memories:

Time Capsule For Me

At any given point in time, I want to be able to recall all of the sights, sounds and emotions the day my daughter entered my life.

I want to see it. I want to have a variety of pictures of Marie's first few minutes in this world. I want to see pictures that show Marie's name written for the first time on the hospital room's dry-erase board, tears running down Wifey's cheeks as she smiled and held our baby girl in her arms, and my little Marie asleep on my chest while I stare up at the ceiling, wondering how I've had two kids in less than two years.

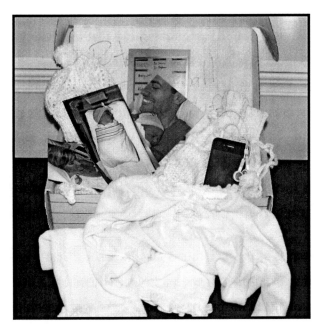

Time capsule

I want to hear it. A twenty-song playlist blared throughout the delivery room, featuring everything from Jay-Z to Katy Perry. And as luck would have it, I was feeling a little unnerved that Rihanna's "S&M" was playing when Marie entered the world, because nothing could make a Dad more frightened for his daughter than associating her with the lyrics, *"...sticks and stones may break my bones, but chains and whips excite me...."*

I want to feel it. When Marie left the hospital, she wore a pink, fluffy outfit, including a cap that had bunny ears sticking straight up, and booties featuring a pair of tiny black eyes, a pink nose, and of course, satin bunny ears. Those are among the things I will collect and keep: printed-out pictures, an MP3 player with her songs, and the bunny suit—the things I can see, hear, and feel from the most incredibly special and amazingly wonderful day that I otherwise wouldn't have been able to remember.

I need to store it. I found an old baseball card box to contain print-outs of the pictures (remember to bring a camera to the hospital), an old iPod™ with headphones to hear Marie's playlist (make sure to include a battery charger), and a Ziploc™ bag to contain her outfit (hey, I'm a guy, it's as cute as I get).

Daddy Letter For My Daughter

On the day Marie was born, I was a mess. We had a false labor the previous day, I had to give a client presentation at work that morning, and our babysitter for Henry bailed on us, causing a last minute scramble. When Marie is old enough, I will share with her the excitement, the anxiety and the fear that was bottled up inside me the day she was born. Every dad is a complete wreck that day, whether he admits or not. After all, you are in a dimly lit, cold hospital room, surrounded by strangers, while your wife is in pain for hours on end, you feel helpless to make her feel better, and all while the best experience in the world is going to happen at any moment.

Looking back on that day, I want my daughter to know that her dad was swearing like a sailor as he fought unprecedented traffic at 9:00 p.m. on the way to the hospital; that her dad nearly missed her birth because he was in the parking lot transferring her brother's car seat to grandpa's car; and that her dad stole a piece of pizza from the hospital floor's community refrigerator. (Give me a break; I hadn't eaten in twelve hours.) And, above all, there are three things I want her to know that I was thinking when I first held her in my arms: boy that pizza was good; how do I make sure she ends up with a good guy like Daddy; and how do I make sure she knows that being smart is cool. These are the types of thoughts, feelings and ideas I will share with my little girl so that she can understand her OCD father a little bit better.

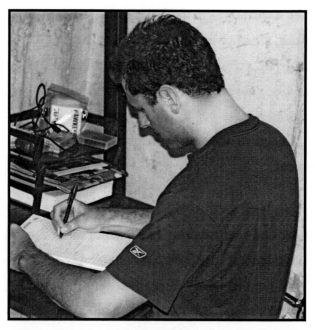

Daddy letter

Daddy Letter For a Son

The idea is the same, although you might be not be inclined to be sweet and sappy for your son. I'd suggest tough love. If it was for my own son, Henry, the three things I would want him to know that I was thinking when I first held him my arms were: do not get a girl pregnant if she's not your wife; the high school quarterback is not God; and you are not entitled to anything, especially not a car on your sixteenth birthday.

Week 1 Recap

Memory is a funny thing. It can't always be trusted, can it? In twenty years, I may not remember the look on my son's face when he first saw me, or that Ne-Yo was the first singer he heard when he entered this world, or how his skin smelled like maple syrup. But, with Marie, not only will I remember what was going on, I'll be able to see it, hear it, and feel it, whenever *WE* want to, together.

WEEK 2: BOND BEFORE IT'S TOO LATE

Professional Baby Pictures; Skin-To-Skin Contact

You've survived the first week, including the three peaceful days in the hospital, post-birth. With the staff who were so polite in answering the basic questions (e.g., "Yes, you are holding the baby perfectly"), so comforting when things don't go smoothly ("It's okay, all babies don't latch right away"), and so helpful when you were too exhausted to move ("Of course I will bring you an extra pillow and blanket"), you just might be hesitant to have to do all of this on your own at home. Those three days were like staying at a hotel, being catered to left and right.

But if the hospital was the calm, then home could be considered the storm, as our first night back home was filled with non-stop hysterical crying that seemed to last for several days. But don't worry, it's okay, it's normal. The first night home with Marie, we found ourselves on our couch at 3:00 a.m., nearing the end of six straight hours of Marie's crying. When I looked at Wifey, I made the mistake of saying, "So, this is why the hospital discharges you on Day 3—once you're home it's too late to give them back." Wifey responded with a frown, muttering, "Yes dear, babies don't come with Nordstrom's 'don't ask, don't tell, we'll take it back whenever, for whatever reason return policy.'" Ouch, that stung.

But Week 2 does get better. In fact, during this week, there will be at least one day that you will actually get more than four hours of sleep, in a row. The panicky parenthood slows down a bit, but that doesn't mean it's time to slack off. You actually have a lot of catching up to do. This is not in terms of cooking, cleaning or other mundane housekeeping duties that you've ignored in lieu of diaper duty; this is in regard to connecting.

Your wife has had a connection with your baby for ten months; you haven't even reached ten days. While this isn't a race with your wife, friendly competition is never a bad thing, especially when it comes to love. I'm not suggesting that your wife has been hogging junior all to herself, but you never got to experience these distinctive bonding moments throughout the various stages of pregnancy:

- The Taut Tummy (First Trimester): Baby is too small to even notice, which causes Mom to keep asking, "Think she's still breathing?"

- The Wiggle Womb (Second Trimester): Baby is bigger and everything from gentle hiccups to baby's own personal Cirque de Soleil event is happening inside Mom's belly.

- The Speedbag Stomach (Third Trimester): Baby is nearing full term and constantly punching and slapping like a Johnson outboard motor.

While this may or may not cause you to be envious, these moments, among others, are how your baby has been bonding with Mommy. And now is the time for you and Baby to connect.

So, the Week 2 message is bond before it's too late. And here are DADspirations to consider doing:

Professional Baby Pictures For Me

I've taken a million pictures in my life, but I would hardly consider myself a photographer. Sure, I will snap the occasional gem, but every other picture seems to capture a closed pair of eyes, someone flipping the bird, or an involuntary muscle twitch of the upper or lower lip. But with a newborn, this should be easy, right? Feed her, burp her, lay her on the bed and click the camera like a maniac. I'm bound to get three pictures out of the lot that are halfway decent, right? Wrong. The lighting made it look like we lived in a dungeon, the shadows made it look like he had one eye, and the angles seemed always to cut off a foot or hand. You don't want someone to ask why she is missing her left ear, do you? Hiring a professional is not cheap, but family and friends usually know someone who is just getting a photography business off the ground, whose work is good enough to show off your infant in style without breaking the bank. Photograph the mandatories first: baby sleeping, baby's toes and baby's fingers. Then get pictures of you and her, her and Wifey and a family shot. Photoshopping yourself into pictures never works. I tried with Henry once and everyone questioned whether he was my own kid or not.

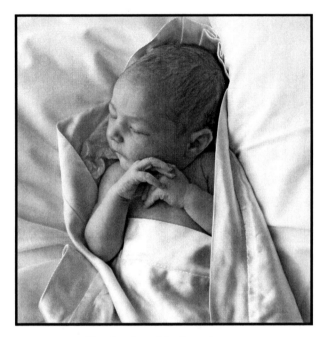

Professional baby picture

Skin-to-Skin Contact For My Daughter

Admit it. Mom went through a lot of crap to give you this baby. For the past year, she's changed her lifestyle, her diet and most importantly her wardrobe. She's not out

clubbing or hanging out at bars; she's been limiting her
fried food and caffeine intake, and her jeans now feature
a woven waistband, for God's sake. Meanwhile, you've
continued to watch *SportsCenter,* eat Cool Ranch Doritos, and drink Miller Lite to your heart's content. Since
mommy got her bonding inside the womb, you're going
to have do yours on the outside. First step is to take your
shirt off. You've been working out this entire time, correct? Me either, but you're in the privacy of your own
home (with the blinds closed, of course), so you're in
good shape as far as your daughter's concerned. She
doesn't care if you're buff. Strip her down to her diaper,
lie on the couch, and place her on your chest. Studies
show that babies are stimulated and comforted by this.
Plus, this provides you with another opportunity you
might be lacking in: sleep. To optimize her introduction
into the art form known as "chillin," manke sure she's
fed, burped, wiped and diaped—you might actually get
an hour of rest out of this.

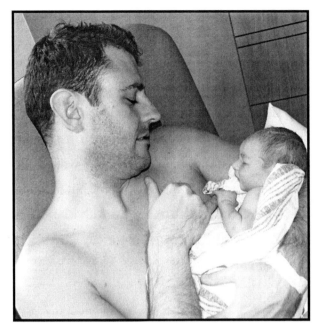

Skin-to-skin contact

Skin-to-Skin Contact For a Son

Don't worry, it doesn't make you less of a man, nor should this freak you out. In fact, this is an excellent opportunity to establish the fundamentals of male bonding at the earliest ages: memorizing and repeating meaningless sports statistics, belching the first half of the alphabet and explaining the art of how to properly navigate the television with a remote control.

Week 2 Recap

Bonding is something we all know is important, but are we always ready for it from the get-go? Newborns know nothing else. They desire it. They crave it. They need it. But for fathers, connecting with their newborns can be a process, if you let it. With Henry, I waited for that connection to happen. It came naturally, but in hindsight, it could have come much sooner. So with Marie, I'm not waiting. This time I'm not letting a day go by without bonding with my little girl.

WEEK 3: BYE, BYE BABY BLUES

Framed Picture; Family and Friends Brunch

The third week of parenthood is known to most as "baby blues" week. It comes right on the heels of two weeks of being in "la-la land" where everything is simply amazing, from baby curling her toes to baby blinking her eyes, and even baby spitting up on Daddy's shirt during Thanksgiving dinner while he was passing the cranberries, in turn, causing him to drop said cranberries on his lap, forcing him to knock the table with his knees, thus spilling red wine in his mashed potatoes, all of which makes him realize that it's only 7:00 p.m., and that he now will spend the rest of the night with a long yellowish-white stain on his dark shirt and a purple-black blotch in the groin area of his khaki pants. But I digress.

The precious first two weeks are dreamlike, a period of time that's more fuzzy than clear, where you seemingly float for fourteen days, never really knowing what time of day it is, whether or not you've showered, what has happened outside of your home, who's seen the baby and who hasn't, and if you've really slept or have just been so tired that you've just thought you slept. Well, this week will quickly bring you back down to Earth from whatever cloud you've been on.

That's because Week 3 is the wake-up call. Dads who maxed out their paternity leave will be going back to work, which means Mom will be at home, with kid, alone, for about eight hours at a time. For us, it was the most stressful week because this gave us the worst thing that can happen to a new dad: time to think.

When I was at work, I wasn't at work. I was thinking.

- How could I just leave them home alone?

- Is Wifey going to be okay without me?

- Will my daughter think that I've abandoned her?

- Am I a horrible husband and father for ditching them or a great husband and father for providing for them?

- Am I going to get fired because I spend more time wondering what they are doing than how to increase my client's product sales?

- If I get fired, would I be able to find a new job?

- If I found a new job, would I still think about being a horrible father?

- Should I have been more prepared so I wouldn't be thinking about them so much?

- Why did we decide to have another child?

As you can see, my OCD is never-ending, but there is a solution. Instead of worrying about how I might mentally damage my newborn before she reaches preschool, I flipped the focus. I couldn't stop myself from thinking, but I could start thinking differently. I decided to celebrate the new family addition instead of worrying about it. And no, I did not just read *The Secret*.

So the Week 3 message is bye, bye baby blues. And here are DADspirations to consider doing:

Framed Picture of My Daughter For Me

It took me three months before I got around to putting up a picture of Henry at work, and when I did, it made me smile every single time I looked at it. I want that same feeling with Marie, so upon returning to work, I didn't waste any time.

Put your daughter on display, but don't feel the need to "CafePress" her onto every single office-related item you can find, such as a calendar, mouse pad, post-it-note pad, iPhone™ case, calculator or shoe horn. This isn't to say she's not beautiful, or you're not proud of her, or that you don't want to show her off, because she is, you are and you do. Just do it tastefully. Your co-workers do not need to see your daughter on the side of a coffee mug during every status report meeting for the next year. Pick out your favorite picture (preferably the lone picture with her eyes open so people know she does in fact have eyes—yes, people do ask that question) and go to your local pharmacy. Spend less than $10 on the frame and keep it simple. There's no need for a frame that features an obnoxious line of copy like "A Star is Born," "Daddy's Little Princess" or "Future Diva." The frame shouldn't take away from the picture of her. It should keep the attention on her. Do you really want to hear someone say, "Diva, huh? She must be a real handful? Well, good luck with that. Oh by the way, she looks like a real cutie." Didn't think so.

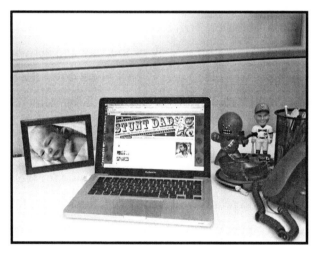

Framed picture

Family and Friends Brunch For My Daughter

Nothing means more to us than family and friends, and nothing is more fun than throwing a party. If you feel the same, why not combine the two and introduce your baby to the people she will come to know and love? I'm not suggesting a Friday night cocktail hour or a Saturday night kegger. Instead, I recommend a chill, relaxed Sunday afternoon brunch, giving people the option to come and go as they please. To make sure this would be all about my baby daughter, and not an excuse for Wifey and me to have Sunday Funday with Bloody Marys, we instituted two rules: any visitor had to a) hold Marie, and b) get their picture taken with her. Why? Because Dad (yes, me) was going to be making a scrapbook of this day and showing it to her when she was older. And twenty years down the road, when Marie will be better acquainted with these same family members and friends, we can look back and see everyone and everything from that special day. In addition to some inevitable laughs, she can always use it as guide for successfully dealing with relatives at family functions in the future. To see that even back then Aunt Tina always tried to be the center of attention by not showing Marie's face as she posed in front of the camera, cousin Mitchell was even then a brat as he pulled on Marie's ear while sporting that toothless smile, and Uncle Larry was a drunk with Marie in one arm and a pint glass full of red wine in the other.

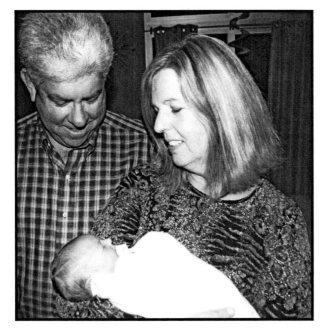

Family and friends brunch

Family and Friends Brunch For a Son

Not much needs to change to apply this to a son, except you might want to ditch the "scrapbook" idea. Instead, collect the pictures and make a video of them. This will have much more of a cool factor for your little dude later in life when any mention of a photo album will have him rolling his eyes, heading for the nearest exit, and looking to go make the latest bad decision with the friends you don't approve of.

Week 3 Recap

Celebrating is subjective. Some scream from the rooftops, some whisper in ears. And, like most things in life, I fall somewhere in the middle of the spectrum. I want to tell, but not shout. I want to hold, but not coddle. I want to love, but not suffocate. Find your happy medium to beat the baby blues that best applies to you.

WEEK 4: CAPTURE THE MOMENTS

Playdates; Monthly Photo Journal

The fourth week of parenthood is a major milestone for several reasons. Your baby is no longer a newborn; he or she will be graduating to infant by the end of the week. Your baby is also starting to react to his or her surroundings. You move to the left, baby's eyes move to the left. You raise your glass of wine in the air and baby's eyes follow. And finally, and I realize I'm going to go out on limb on this one so forgive me if I'm being presumptuous, you've managed to avoid smothering, dropping or throwing said baby for an entire month. For that, you deserve a huge CONGRATULATIONS! That is no easy feat, my friend!

On a more serious note, you've likely noticed some major changes with baby. Baby has started to coo, grunt and hum, which, hopefully, will bring out your inner silliness and you'll start mastering the goo-goos and gah-gahs as you interact with your little one. Our own little one has also gone from looking like Benjamin Button to someone who is starting to showcase family features:

- She has Mom's nose! That is, the soft, adorable little curved nose instead of Daddy's big, honking schnoz.

- She has Grandma's eyes, the piercing blue eyes that are judging every word you say and every action you do!

- She has Grandpa's smile—the wide, brimming smile that is absent any teeth!

- She has Daddy's ears! Ugh. The big, clunky ears will have us begging her to keep her hair long enough to cover them.

- And she also has Daddy's feet! Great, she has big ears and big feet, which can only mean she's going to have a big…purse.

Lots of changes are happening with baby, both physically and mentally. And unless you plan accordingly, it's easy to miss them. Now is the time to enjoy observing everything that is happening with her. You've seen the movie *Gorillas in the Mist,* haven't you? It's gonna be a lot like that. I even bought a fog machine. And I'll be damned if any poachers are gonna get to MY baby!

So, the Week 4 message is capture the moments. And here are DADspirations to consider doing:

Schedule Playdates For Me

It's sometimes hard to think outside of your four walls during that first month of parenthood. With Henry, leaving the house during the first few months was more out of necessity than by choice: doctor's appointments, grocery stores and family birthdays, but the newness of it all can consume you and you can easily go through four weeks forgetting that there is life beyond baby. Who knew there is more to parenthood than to swaddle baby, soothe tantrums and change diapers?

You owe it to your child to urge interaction with other children, even at the infant stage, because it ultimately forces you to interact with other parents. Sure, it's ador-able to watch infants sit there and stare at each other and drool, but this is just as much for you, for two reasons: 1) it sets the foundation for years to come; and 2) to learn tips and tricks.

Now is the time to start researching which local kids you want your child to hang out with for the next few years, and the best way to determine that is through the parents. Shockingly, parents are no strangers to cliques: from the cool kids to the pot smokers to the nerds, all seemingly gravitate to one another ten to fifteen years after gradua-tion. So, unless you find the families who share the same values and morals as you and your wife, you could end up with the kids who are destined for detention hall and careers of manual labor. Of course, this may not bother you if you were the kid who pulled fire alarms and stole cars in junior high.

Not sure how to meet parents? Check online to see what playgroups exist that match up with your interests. One excellent source for this can be found at www.meet-up.com. You can type in 'playgroups' in the Topic or Interest field as well as your ZIP code. Chances are good that you'll receive a slew of opportunities. If you aren't the online type, then I'd recommend grabbing your kid, some fresh baked cookies, and start knocking on the doors of homes in your neighborhood which have a minivan in the driveway. Below are some quick reminders on what separates the trustworthy parents from the suspect parents.

- **Trustworthy parents:** They arrive with and pick up their child on time; they offer to bring you or the kids treats or offer to help clean up; they say positive things about their spouse; they ask more than three questions about your background; they have no rips or tears in their clothing. *Bottom line: they are people you don't run from in public.*

- **Suspect parents:** You have to call or beg the parent to pick up their child; their child wears the same dirty clothes to every playdate; they repeatedly ask to take leftover food home with them; they never offer to host; they reek of smoke, fast food, and ethanol—the leftover smell from an apparent long night of binge drinking; and they complain about their lazy and unaffectionate partner.

Bottom line: you would rather saw your arm off than leave your kid alone with any of them for five minutes.

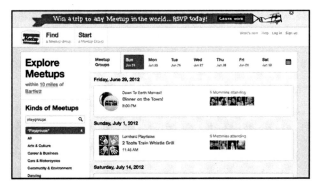

Setting up playdates

Monthly Photo Journal For My Daughter

You will take a million pictures during baby's first couple of years, maybe even two million. You will have pictures of baby sitting, standing, crawling, walking, laughing, crying and countless other actions. However, the one thing our son's photos didn't include was growing. Sure, scanning through iPhoto, I see it has all of our pictures organized by date that could reflect our son's evolution, but it lacks a monthly consistency that would have been nice to capture. April pictures would show him bundled up in a blanket; May would show him sleeping in his cradle; June would show him spread eagle on the quilt that your wife's college roommate's mom made, and so forth. But with Marie, it was important to me to have a more structured approach so that she'd be able to look back on these pictures and have her own personal visual timeline.

On her monthly birthday until she is two years old, we are taking photos using the following criteria:

1. Awake: I've said this before, but open eyes prove to the world that your baby is alive and well. Take it from me, it's embarrassing when friends and family looks at a picture of your baby whose eyes are closed and they poke the picture in an attempt to see movement.

2. Looking directly at the camera: Show off that pretty face! Seeing half a face every few months might raise some eyebrows: Black eye? Bad cut? Abnormal growth? Time to call DCFS (Department of Children and Family Services)?

3. Wearing the same onesie*: Similar to the picture frame idea in Week 2. Put her in a plain pink creeper;

keep the focus on baby's development, not on the parent's personal style preferences. Sorry, flannel lovers, it's not cute—even on a newborn.

4. Same spot*: Get 'em in the same chair with her favorite stuffed animal, so you can see how baby gets bigger and bigger in that rocker and Peggy the Pig becomes smaller and smaller.

5. Same time of day and month*: Snap in the afternoon with sunny, natural light. Consistency is key and it keeps you from slacking off—having one or two pictures with a night background or thinking you can Photoshop your way out of missing Month 6 will only cause regret and anguish.

   Requires foresight.

Monthly Photo Journal For a Son

Two minor changes and you should be good to go. 1) Make sure to switch the pink onesie to blue; and 2) No little boy wants his picture taken alongside a stuffed pig.

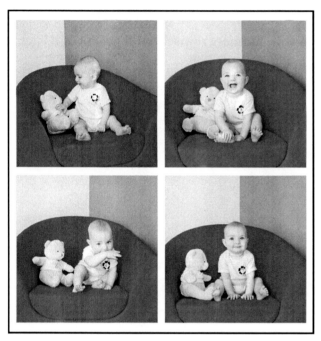

Monthly photo journal

Week 4 Recap

As you know by now, aside from feeding and burping, you've spent a lot of time watching your baby. Baby is exploring, noticing that he or she, hopefully, has two arms, both legs, and ten fingers and toes, but isn't really able to control them. The first month is a major marker to the rest of your baby's milestones. So now is the time to start planning and thinking ahead. The more work you put in now, the more reward you'll get out of it later, and so will your child.

MONTH 2

WEEK 5: SHOW THE LOVE

Spa Certificate; Pearl

The first month of parenthood is behind you. Those couple of days in the hospital seem like a lifetime ago, and by now, you and your wife have likely established a solid routine. If your wife is breastfeeding, this means you get to sleep from 10:00 p.m.-6:00 a.m. while she nurses throughout the night. If your baby is on formula, this means you could be making bottles in the wee hours

of the night (and sleepwalking at least once into the bedroom door while making the formula run). Either way,
when morning comes, you are getting out of that house
as fast as humanly possible.

But once you're at the office, it's easy to immerse
yourself into the joys of TPS reports (Testing Proce-
dure Specification), broken copy machines and some
co-worker showing you his "O-face," all the while forgetting that your wife is home, alone, feeding baby every
three hours, consoling baby every two hours, and imag-
ining every single hour what it would be like to take a
shower this week—just once—this week.

I'm not saying your wife is going to become a caged
animal who can't leave her pen and start hysterically
jumping onto furniture or act like a rat who's completely
boxed in and slamming her head against your bedroom
wall. However, if she's been indoors all during the month
of December (when, for us Midwesterners, the ground
looks like the Hoth system and the skies look like something out of a Terminator movie), then, for her sake and
yours, it's time to get her out of the house. Encourage her
to do something alone, something girly, something that
will give her peace, quiet and comfort.

And, while you're experiencing this newfound joy of making sure your Number One, your wife, is taken care of, make sure your Number Two, your infant, gets taken care of as well. Now is the perfect time to start another project for your baby girl. For you parents who are already tired of projects for your children, here is your first and only WAKE-UP CALL. I'm giving you this because if you feel life is starting to become all about your daughter, then guess what? WELCOME TO PARENTHOOD. I hope you got YOU out of your system before you decided to bring a child into this world, because for the next twenty years, it isn't all about you anymore. The sooner you realize that and accept it, the happier your life will be. But I digress, again.

While Momma's gift will be immediate, my daughter's gift will be annual, for the next eighteen years. This project could be something that you and your little one can make together, something that you can make a day out of, something that will last a lifetime. You need to show appreciation to the two most important people in your life, because both of them deserve it.

So the Week 5 message is show the love. And here are DADspirations to consider doing:

Spa Certificate For Mom (which is also for me)

Whether your wife is a reflector, an inner discoverer, or a get-me-out-of-the-houser, sending her to a local spa for a few hours will rejuvenate her as a woman, wife, and mother. I promise you, this will score you more husband points than when you bought her Arby's Roast Beef and Cheddar at 4:00 a.m. during her pregnancy cravings. But don't be afraid of terms such as 'European Conditioning Facial,' 'Deep Tissue Massages' or 'Mud Bath.' Know your budget, walk into the spa, and they will take care of the rest. To put a little icing on the cake, you can put the spa certificate into a nice card along with a wallet-sized favorite picture of your wife and baby together. This way, she can still have a part of her daughter with her while she's away and can always have a little something to remind her of the special afternoon you gave her.

While this seems like it's all about Mom (and you should tell her that it is, several times, over and over, multiple times a day, for hours on end, until the day you die), you'll get alone time with your baby, which for me, was the first time I had her all to myself. Read her a book, give her tummy time on the activity mat, or introduce her to the art of watching Bob Ross or Kung Fu. Imagine a Sunday afternoon that looks like this: a) Mom alone, spa, champagne; and b) Dad, daughter, couch, beer. It's a win-win for the whole family.

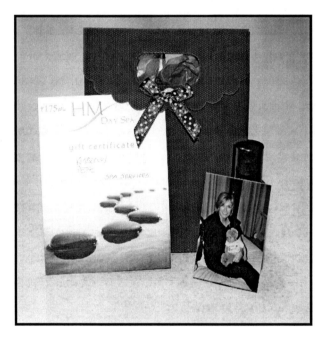

Spa certificate

Pearl For My Daughter

This is a small gift that becomes large over time, a gift that will take a few years for her to comprehend. It's a gift that after eighteen years will remind her of why she'll always be Daddy's little girl and possess a magical deflector shield so that no boy, guy or dude will talk, touch or even look in her direction until she is thirty-five, maybe forty, years of age. This gift is a pearl. And every year, on the same date, I'll give another pearl to my daughter. And it's going to be our day, whether she is six years old and I take her out to Barney's Ice Cream Hut or she is twelve years old and I take her shopping at the mall. This day will be something that we share, just the two of us. And when she's eighteen, we'll go to a local jeweler and have the pearls strung any way she wants them. There are many ways to wear pearls, and whether it's a pearl necklace (get your mind of the gutter), a pearl collar (no seriously, get it out of the gutter) or a pearl choker (really, even this makes you snicker?), I want that decision to be hers. I want her decision to reflect her style, her personality and her attitude when that special day comes (oh, come on now!).

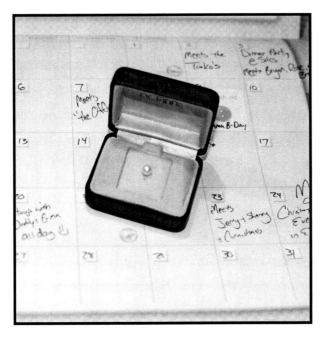

Pearl for my daughter

Pearl For a Son

ABORT! ABORT! No self-respecting father would give his son pearls to make a necklace. There is so much wrong with that on so many levels that I won't even think about how that might potentially be acceptable. Instead, give him a watch. Start him on a Mickey Mouse watch and evolve the gift as he ages, ending with a Petak Philippe watch when he graduates from college. Get him in the habit early of wearing it on a regular basis. By the time he's ready for grammar school, not only will he have learned how to tell time, but when he needs to be home by 5:00 p.m. for dinner, he won't be able to use the excuse, "Sorry Dad, I didn't know what time it was."

Week 5 Recap

Show the love and the love will be returned, immediately or down the road. Take care of the woman who made you happier than ever and the baby who made you realize that you could cherish someone with the same intensity as you feel for your wife. But remember to have fun with it. When Wifey comes back from the spa, brag to her how excited your baby got when Bob Ross painted a happy little squirrel next to a waterfall or when David Carradine drop-kicked a group of bad guys. (Honey, that's going to be our little girl, fending off any would-be suitors with her mad ninja skills). Or, when purchasing her first pearls, include a picture of the two of you and see how much the two of you change over the years. See how as she gets prettier and prettier, you get… wiser and wiser.

WEEK 6: FOSTER GROWTH

Our First Events; Planting a Tree

Six weeks in, you've probably experienced your baby's first smile, watched him or her track your face from side to side, and received the first of many golden showers to come. And don't think just because you have a girl that you're off the hook when it comes to the yellow fountain of youth. I learned the hard way when, after Wifey warned me, I casually let my guard down while changing Marie's diaper, and subsequently, received a liquid stream of consciousness from her.

Aside from that humbling experience, you will finally start to see some action out of baby. I know that sounds bad, but come on, let's face it, you honestly couldn't tell the difference between still photographs of your baby or any three-minute video of her up to this point; ninety percent of both our kids' pictures highlight them in one of three places: on their back, on their belly, or on the boob. No, I'm not trying to compare their first four weeks to a Skinemax soft-porn movie.

Instead of being that adorable, blinking, little lump of yours, he or she will start to bloom. Some things to look for:

- Flattened hands: Gone are the days when you were convinced she was going to be the next Laila Ali with her clenched fists. The hands actually open and close now, if only to grab anything within reaching distance. Good thing we just let the ladies wear the hoop earrings, right fellas?

- Flailing arms: Contrary to what you might have thought, she's not a doll; the kid actually does move, even though she might resemble a fish out of water.

- Clapping: She won't have the synchronization down pat yet, but every once in a while her hands will come together and you'll feel an irresistible urge to start singing "Kumbaya."

While he or she is starting to grow, so is your family. Mom is getting more comfortable with her role as the boss and you're settling into your role for the rest of your lifetime as second-in-command. Between baby's mental development and physical growth, now is the optimal time to start documenting all of it.

So, the Week 6 message is to foster growth, and here are DADspirations to consider doing:

Our First Events For Me

For Henry, we have all the major milestones written down: first smile, laugh, sleeps through the night, sits up, crawls, yadda, yadda, yadda…While those are all warm fuzzies and make you feel extra special nice inside, I'm going to go the extra mile with Marie by adding some additional firsts that even BabyCenter doesn't have on its website. There is one thing that babies and dads have in common—chilling. And all dads know that the best place to chill out is on the couch in front of the television. Since Marie is a rockstar at lying in my arms for extended periods of time, I'm going to start writing down each of the firsts we share together on

TV, seeing as how she's a little too young to take to live events:

- **1st Sporting Event—Chicago Blackhawks vs. Detroit Red Wings:** I documented the game with a picture of us in our swag (onesie for her, Winter Classic Throwback jersey for me, a newspaper clipping of the box score (Hawks win 3-2!), noting the number of times I caught myself swearing at the referee (more than my age), and the type, but not the amount, of beer I drank (Miller Lite, classy!).

- **1st Concert—The Killers:** I documented the show with a picture of us in band t-shirts (AC/DC for her, Van Halen for me), wrote down the song list (noting their stellar encore rendition of "Human"), purchased an MP3 download of the show (so that I can play it to her at night when she's going to sleep), and the type, but not the amount, of liquor I drank (tequila on the rocks).

- **1st Animated Movie—*The Little Mermaid:*** I documented the flick with a picture of us in our cartoon pajamas (Kung Fu Panda sleeper for her,

Avengers t-shirt for me), purchased a stuffed toy from the movie (every girl needs an Ariel), permanently borrowed the DVD from Blockbuster (only cost me $10) and the type, but not the amount, of wine I drank (box wine from Target).

- **1st Restaurant—Johnny's Taco Hut:** Sure, chilling in front of the television rocks, but you do have to get out of the house once in a while. I documented the eatery with a picture of us (well, Wifey and me) wearing sombreros, noting what kind of food we ate (uh, tacos), what compliments Marie received ("Dude, she's got really big eyes."), grabbed a matchbook for a keepsake (romantic, aren't I?), and the type, but not the amount, of margaritas we drank (mango, strawberry, and classic).

- **1st State Line—Illinois/Wisconsin:** I documented the trip with a picture of us under the Welcome to Wisconsin sign (in two feet of snow), where we were going (our lake house), when we first wanted to turn back (ten minutes into the car ride), what the highlight of the trip was (Marie cooing while Daddy made a fire), and the type, but not the amount, of soda we drank in the car (fountain Coke and Squirt).

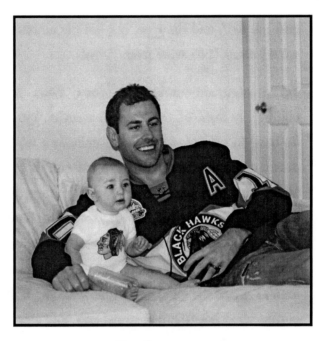

Our first events

Planting a Tree For My Daughter*

I'm not a big environmentalist, I don't have a garden, and only sometimes do I recycle. But planting a tree for Marie will not only give us shade, produce oxygen, and all that good stuff, it'll also be something that she'll always have, see, and touch as they both grow. And, as you've likely caught on to by now, it will be great to take annual pictures to see the progression of growth.

And then, twenty years from now, when Marie will likely tower over me, Big Wood will be towering over both of us. An added bonus is that this gift requires no money (find a local nursery that's looking to give trees away to clear inventory), requires no intensive labor (dig hole, drop tree, done), and requires no maintenance (thank you Mother Nature). But remember, the type of land-scape tree will also mystically indirectly influence the type of girl you raise:

- **Magnolia:** Girly Girl - Exceptional beauty, fragrant, pinkish-white bloom.

- **Apple:** Girl Next Door - Nothing says farmer's daughter better.

- **Dogwood:** Bipolar Girl - Blooms in both spring and fall. That's just downright crazy.

- **Maple:** Sporty Girl - Blooms in fall, which is the only season where the Big 4 overlap (football, baseball, hockey, and basketball).

- **Spruce:** Bitchy Girl - Contains prickly needles. Say no more, unless you're into that kind of thing.

- **Birch:** Nerdy Girl - Better known for its bark than its leaves. How lame is that?

- **Oak:** Cool Girl - Tallest, strongest, boldest badass tree on the planet.

Because Marie was born in November, this idea had to wait until April when it was a better time for planting a maple tree.

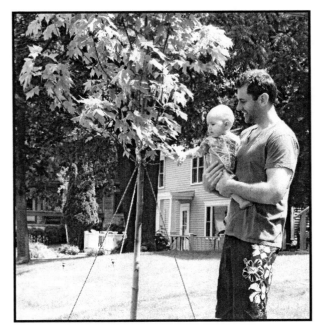

Planting a tree

Planting a Tree For a Son

This one is definitely universal, and even the type of tree you decide to plant aligns with what type of boy you raise. However, I would shy away from a magnolia tree, as Girly Boy doesn't have the same appeal, unless you're a die-hard Shirley MacLaine, Olympia Dukakis and Sally Field fan. In that case, I'd recommend that you stop having any more children, and start saving now for trips to the psychiatrist during your son's adolescent years.

Week 6 Recap

Exciting times are ahead and pretty soon, your baby will be a walkin' talkin', jumpin' jivin' little person and if you don't start documenting now, you'll wish you had. It's easy to "skip that one," "I'll get the next one," or "I'll write it down later," but chances are it will become a distant memory if you don't. Keep things handy; have a plan and stick to it: think it, record it and execute it.

WEEK 7: EXPRESSION THROUGH MUSIC

Memorize Lullabies; Dedicate a Song

It's Week 7, also known as (in my best Chris Berman voice) PRIME TIME! As in learning. This is because baby's brain will grow five centimeters by the end of Month 3, which, for non-Europeans, is two inches. Doesn't sound like much? Well, here are a few things that measure two inches: a sugar packet, your thumb, or what happens due to cold water shrinkage!

Now, measure two inches against your baby's head and suddenly you realize there is going to be a lot of room to fill with the most important of information. And what can be more important than . . . your voice? Textures, shapes, and all the touchy-feely stuff is great, but if I could have my baby girl know one thing right now, it would be my voice. The more she hears my voice, the more comfortable with me she will be. So when I explain to her why the Chicago Bulls simply cannot let me down as much as the Chicago Bears did, she'll just sit there and smile. When I want to rant how Facebook seriously needs to stop making all of these non-changeable changes, she will giggle. And, above all else, when I sing to her, she will sleep. Immediately. For hours on end. Okay, I'll take just a few hours—three blissfully quiet hours. Hell, I'd even be happy with two hours.

Yes, it's true, I'm a fraud. Behind all the good intentions I have for my daughter, my deepest, darkest secret for wanting to talk to her is so that she will sleep, which in turn, will let me sleep. Sue me. I'd prefer to think I'm improving our means of communication: the more I talk, the quicker she falls asleep, although it's more like a boredom-induced coma.

So, the Week 7 message is expression through music, and here are DADspirations to consider doing:

Memorize Lullabies

Don't groan, this will take an hour tops. These are not novels that you need to memorize. Why lullabies instead of just one lullaby? Because singing "Bye, baby bunting" over and over for an hour will drive you to grab an ice pick and jab it into your own ear. You will need options, for your own sanity and your wife's too. You think she actually likes to hear a god-awful singer sing a god-awful song? And you might be wondering, why lullabies instead of your favorite songs? For a simple reason: lullabies were developed for people who cannot sing, which I can't, and neither can you. Go ahead, ask your wife. She'll tell you, "nails on a chalkboard." Lullabies are short, soothing rhymes to force your infant into submission, er ..., sleep. They are not for *American Idol* auditions. I'm not Michael Buble. I'm not Michael Bolton (thank God). Hell, I'm not even Michael McDonald. So, as tempted as I might be to try turning "Yah Mo B There" into a lullaby, I won't, for Wifey's sake and for Marie's sake. Whether it's "Twinkle, Twinkle Little Star" or "Silent Night," take sixty minutes out of your life and learn four lullabies. And then, just to prove you still have an ounce of creativity at your age, make up one additional lullaby, using my four-step process below:

- **Think:** What do I want to tell my daughter? It's got to have a good message to her, not just a load of crappy words that make my wife look at me and question, "What the hell did you just say to her?"

- **Write:** Twelve lines, rhyming, with rhythm. It's like poetry (gulp). No, it's like rap (wahoo!), just soft-sounding rap.

- **Tune:** I have no musical abilities. I'm tone deaf, so I'm going to cheat number 4 by stealing, er …, borrowing a tune from another lullaby. Thank you, "Hush Little Baby." You might want to do something similar.

- **Lull:** Put it all together and release my inner Johannes Brahms. (Dude, this doesn't mean use a German accent, just that he was a famous composer.)

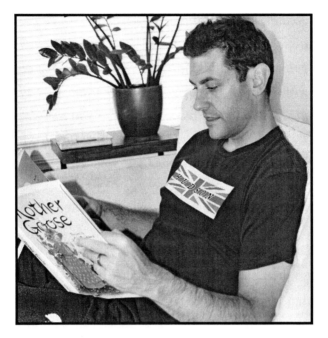

Memorize lullabies

Dedicating a Song For a Daughter

After the hard work is done with the lullaby, it's time to get sappy. I don't mean calling up the local light FM radio station and requesting they play a love song in honor of your little girl and call it a night. I can hear it now:

To the 3-month old Marie Densmore, we've got a special request from your daddy. Even though you can't possibly fathom what I am saying or why I am saying it, your daddy wanted us to play a Whitney Houston song for you tonight. Without further ado, to his baby girl, love Dad. Here is... "I Will Always Love You."

Excuse me while I go heave in the bathroom.

Instead of causing radio listeners to snicker at your epic failure to achieve Super Dad status, I'm talking about creating something that will be long-lasting as well as cool, a song that will always be associated with just her and you. Pick out a song that can be played at some of her special lifetime moments, such as her baptism, a road trip to Grandma's, and her wedding day. Unless you want to permanently damage her psyche, that rules out some classics, such as "Welcome to the Jungle" and "Thunderstruck," but it leaves the door open for some lighter favorites from U2 or Jason Mraz. Whatever the song, have fun with it. When she's old enough to appreciate it, give her a handmade frame containing the songs lyrics as a gift. Or, when she's old enough to know that it's not cool to hang with you, but still young enough to want to, spend a Friday night with her, eating popcorn, drinking milk-shakes and conducting a song-a-thon, seeing how many times you can play it over and over until one of you turns it off. No matter what you do to further the bond, plan on playing it often enough for her to give you a wink later on in life when it randomly plays overhead while you two are getting a coffee at Starbucks (or whatever replaces coffee as the "it" thing to drink in 2032).

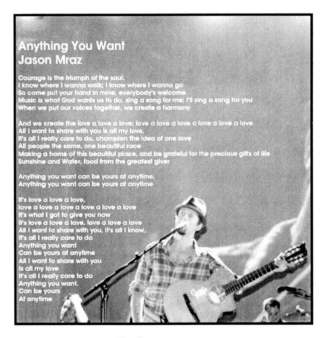

Dedicate a song

Dedicating a Song For a Son

The shackles are off on this one, Dad. No artist off-limits, no genre forbidden. Snoop, Garth, Marley, Clapton, Plant, Garfunkel, Axel. Doesn't matter. Whatever you choose, play it loud, and play it proud: on the way to his little league games, when you're making Sunday pancakes, and at his bachelor party. If it has the word 'fire' in it, even better, because we all know boys and men of all shapes, ages and sizes share a common love for fire.

Week 7 Recap

While she won't be engaging in conversation with me just yet, my wish is that hearing my voice will bring her comfort and familiarity the more I sing to her. Hopefully, her first words won't be, "Stop singing, Daddy," but I'll stay optimistic for now. Keep in mind, the real reason behind all of this singing is to get her to sleep as soon as humanly possible.

WEEK 8: DON'T HANG YOUR HEAD

Date Night; Favorite Book

You have lasted another month, and everyone is still alive and well (presumably). Another CONGRATULA-TIONS is in order. I'm sure things on the parenthood front are smooth sailing by now; however, I'm willing to bet that the quality alone time between you and your wife has reached an all-time low. After all, the past eight weeks, or 1,440 hours, or 86,400 minutes, or 5,184,000 seconds have been mostly about your new addition to the family and not much about the two people who brought junior(ette) into the world. Your life has been about wipin' and diapin' baby's behind, and not tappin' and pattin' Wifey's behind.

Several reasons could account for the lack of husband and wife time:

- **No time:** Husband works ten hours a day, wife works twenty-four hours a day. Do the math.

- **No energy:** If you both happen to have an over-lapped thirty minutes of free time, the race to bed is for sleep, not for nookie.

- **No money:** No, I'm not suggesting money should be exchanged for sex in your house. I was actually referring to the increased spending now that baby is in the world, which also increases stress and decreases any desire for romance.

- **No hand:** Whoever has the upper hand in the rela-tionship also controls the extracurricular activities, and—trust me—you won't have it.

- **No interest:** Parenthood has made you lazy, and going to a gym is likely the furthest thing from your mind, well—a close second, to sex.

This is not one of the happiest times of parenthood, but there is no denying the reality of it. I hate to be the one to break it to you, but life is not all sunshine and rainbows. There are going to be some days, weeks and months where you might question what you've gotten yourself into. You will argue with your wife about where cooking utensils should go; you will get frustrated with your infant for not pooping when she needs to poop; and you will get pissed off at yourself for not rising above it all. It's incredibly difficult not to sweat the small stuff and it's impossible to avoid challenging situations and annoying moments. It's going to happen.

However, there are things you can do to counterbalance some of the not-so-fun stuff. You can rekindle the passion. You can express your warmth. Or you can follow the advice from Sylvester Stallone in *Rocky 5:*

> *...It ain't about how hard ya hit. It's about how hard you can get hit and keep moving forward. But ya got to be willing to take the hits, and not pointing fingers saying you ain't where you wanna be because of him, or her, or anybody! Cowards do that and that ain't you! You're better than that!*

So, the Week 8 message is don't hang your head. And here are DADspirations to consider doing:

Date Night For Me (and Wifey)

Yes, you owe this to your wife. She went through nine months of labor, increases in waist sizes, and could have an infant hanging off her boob for several hours a day. Taking her out for a night on the town is the least you can do. You should do something a little special, something out of the ordinary, as a reminder that you are more than just two people raising a baby (this means not going to any restaurants that have the words "Value Meal" on the menu). With that in mind, here are a few things to avoid:

- Taking her to a movie where you sit in the dark, don't speak for two hours, and both fall asleep before anything good happens.

- Hitting up a bar where you'll have way too many drinks, end up arguing about who would have to wake up at 3:00 a.m. to feed the baby, and you both fall asleep before anything good happens.

- Taking her to (what used to be) your favorite restaurant where you'll end up over-analyzing the price of the meal, second-guessing whether you can afford dessert, and, again, you both fall asleep before anything good happens.

Instead, plan to do NOTHING. No reservations. No commitments. No agenda. Once your babysitter arrives, give him or her a high-five, head out the door, and spend the next three hours doing whatever happens to draw your interest. If you feel active, go ice-skating. If you feel lazy, sit in a park and talk. If you get horny, find an alley. For those 180 minutes, just be that couple, doing whatever you used to do as 'just a couple,' and enjoying the freedoms that come with being 'just a couple.'

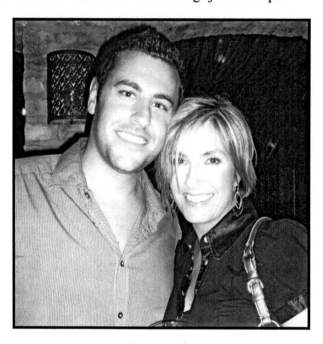

Date night

Read Favorite Book For My Daughter

I'm not talking about the latest board book from Sandra
Boynton or one of Mother Goose's nursery rhymes. This
is about your favorite book, the book you've read more
times than you can remember, the book you recommend
when a friend or co-worker is desperate for a sugges-
tion. This is the book that your little girl will identify you
with, for better or for worse. So choose wisely, because
there are pros and cons to each choice. Since there is no
perfect answer, the question boils down to what values
are you willing to sacrifice for your daughter? Whatever
your choice, your daughter will get to know who you are
through this book, whether she ends up liking what she
finds out or not. Here is what your choice can say about
you:

- **Classic:** You're a traditionalist, a stickler for rules,
  and will stay up late waiting for her to come home.

- **Comedy:** You're emotional, the person she turns
  to for a good laugh or cry; you are flexible with
  discipline but a sucker when your daughter bats her
  eyelashes.

- **Adventure:** You're a thrill seeker, never happy with the status quo and always in search of the next best thing. This means you're daughter will likely travel the world, avoid corporate America, and settle down in an Indonesian village teaching English to the native children.

- **Drama:** You're the serious type. You don't take guff and she respects you, but she will also hate you until she graduates from college, until she realizes that you made a real woman out of her.

- **Tragedy:** You're lonely and sad, dress in blacks and grays, and are generally an unhappy person, yet she knows you'll be there with chocolate and Diet Coke when she comes to you with the love triangle she has found herself in.

- **Mystery:** You're viewed as a problem she can't solve: either you are never home or always changing your mind, and these are not good things.

- **Romance:** You're a confused individual, and she will likely end up questioning your manhood.

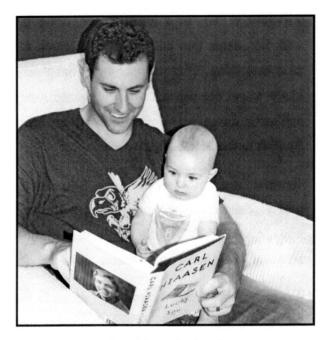

Read favorite book

Read Favorite Book For a Son

Nothing to change much here; reading is universal. But remember, it's man-to-man time now. If you read *Jane Eyre* to your daughter (and if it's your favorite book, please don't admit this to your buddies), I'd recommend something a little more in the guy department. If you are struggling for the *Die Hard* of novels, head over to your local library and pick out a Jack Higgins or Clive Cussler book. These books pull elements from all of the above, which in my view, makes you one badass hero of a dad.

Week 8 Recap

After two months, remember that if your child is a girl you have two girls in your life: mom and daughter. If you thought it was difficult to please one, then you will be hard-pressed to appease another one. But you can do it. Like any other challenge in life, apply yourself the best you can and life will usually end up being okay. Take Wifey wherever works best for you two and read to your daughter whatever resonates most with you. Take care of them both and they'll take care of you.

MONTH 3

WEEK 9: TEACHING IS BELIEVING

Girls' Night Out; Dance With Daughter

By now, some of you might be telling your family, friends, and co-workers that your baby is sleeping through the night—which is a complete and utter lie. But if it makes you feel better to say that, go right ahead! I don't consider five or six hours "sleeping through the night," because even if the baby goes to bed at midnight, you're still getting up before the sun does. There is no loophole, no 'kind of' or 'sort of.' You are just like the rest of us tired, sleep-deprived parents, and we resent you for even trying to suggest you might have had even ONE decent night's sleep in the past two months. When she starts sleeping from 7:00 p.m. to 7:00 a.m., then you can proudly and honestly brag how you have the best sleeper in the world. Phew, now I feel better.

On a more positive note, you can probably tell that your little one is responding more and more to the sound of your voice. It's pretty neat to see Marie's eyes ping-pong back and forth when Wifey and I have a conversation, or argue over how we are going to afford daycare, disagree about which groceries we need to buy, contend about when we are going to buy a house, bicker as to where we are moving, feud over when we are going to get a minivan, dispute whether we should get a dog, hash out whose turn it is to feed the baby, hassle over making dinner, quibble over doing the laundry, wrestle over washing the dishes, lock horns over taking out the trash, squabble about who's shoveling the driveway, starting a *mêlée* over making Henry's lunches for the week, who's pulling their weight and who's not ... and yep, I think that it's it. Sorry, it's been a tough week. :-)

I feel that raising kids sometimes requires an instruction manual, even though we just went through all this with Henry twenty months ago, because any hope for structure and planning seem impossible to make and keep. But if you can't tell by now, I'm an optimist!

So, the Week 9 message is that teaching is believing. And here are DADspirations to consider doing:

Schedule a Girls' Night Out For Wifey (and Me)

Last week was about you and Wifey spending time together, but this week you should remind her that she has some very close friends that she hasn't been able to spend quality time with for over two months. Even though she might protest, insist that she take some 'friend time,' and do not take no for an answer. I don't presume to know your wife or what your wife may or may not enjoy doing with her friends, so for this one you might have to figure out the details on your own. I know, the thought is pretty scary, but I have faith in you.

I know you're probably thinking: "What's in it for me?" Well, you get to have a happy wife, which translates to a happy life. Plus, I got to watch a *Star Wars* movie marathon from 7:00 p.m. to 2:00 a.m. So don't blow it. To give you some initial ideas, here is what I did. Fortunately, my parents live twenty minutes away, so I took the kids to their house on a Saturday night, and left Wifey with the following itinerary for the evening:

- Take the longest shower you've ever had and sing as loud as you want.

- Take as long as you want to blow dry your hair, paint your nails, and put on make-up.

- Wear the sexiest dress you have, including the C.F.M. boots that bring out the tiger in you. Meow.

- A limo will pick you up at 7:30 p.m. sharp, accompanied by your favorite peeps and a bottle of champagne.

- Drink multiple glasses of wine at the pre-dinner lounge bar and flirt with the waiter if you feel so inclined.

- Enjoy all the raw fish you can eat at the hip new sushi restaurant.

- Have a shot or two or three at the nightclub you girls go to and shake your tailfeathers.

- Sleep-in (alone, please) as late as you want and enjoy the pot of coffee that is set to start brewing at 10:00 a.m.

- Read the newspaper, eat a wonderful breakfast, and take a nap before we come home after lunch.

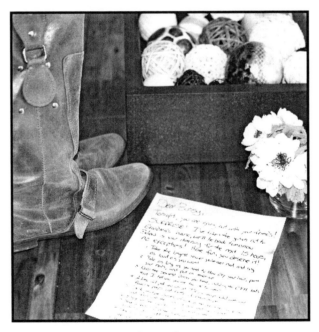

Girls' night out

Teaching Dancing For My Daughter

Like many parents, we want our daughter to be graceful, feel elegant and show poise, so what better way to do that than by teaching Marie how to dance? A short-term bonus: she's small enough to where I'll be carrying her for a couple of years and won't step on any toes. For an added bonus, practicing now will make me less of a clown on her wedding day when we dance to the song I picked out in Week 7. And while I'm no Fred Astaire, I'm no Fred Flintstone, either. And I can prepare myself ahead of time for the various styles and stages of dancing that await me:

- **The Waltz** (1st year): We'll start easy, as this will require the least amount of practice for me: she'll be snuggled up with me in my arms, and my attention will be on avoiding the coffee table and the rocking chair.

- **The Ballroom** (toddler years): My baby girl will probably channel her inner Disney Princess and want to act very prim and proper around the family room after we have our evening tea party.

- **The Freestyle** (elementary years): I have two nieces, and if they're any measure, I can expect complete and utter awesomeness, consisting of twirling, flailing of arms, lots of jumping, and a pretty decent workout.

- **The Swing** (teenage years): Dancing with me will probably be considered lame, so if I'm going to drag her to the dance floor, I'll at least be sure to keep things upbeat with lots of turns, twists and dips.

- **The Ghost** (college years): Who are we kidding? She'll be at college and I'll be lucky even to see her during the holidays, so I'll either dance in my head or grab one of her old stuffed animals and think about all of her toes I had stepped on over the years.

- **The Dance** (Wedding Day): This will be the culmination of dancing with her all of my life, the moment where I weep internally at losing her to some guy who's not good enough for her, but also the moment where I can show off my fancy footwork from all of the years practicing with her.

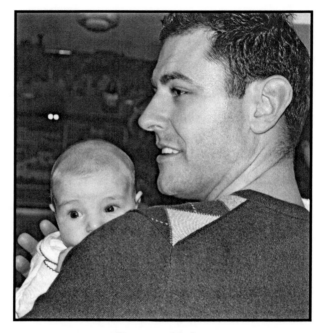

Dance with her

Teaching Dancing For a Son

It's okay to teach your son to dance, if you don't mind seeing him in a leotard when he becomes a teenager. Instead of dancing, I'd recommend taking junior over to the local pool and getting him used to the water. Start teaching him the fundamentals of swimming. However, just because he was "in a pool" for the previous ten months, I wouldn't start teaching him how to hold his breath under water just yet.

Week 9 Recap

My advice for the two favorite girls in your life: spoil them! This is not for any other reason than it's just fun. Your wife will love the time she gets to spend with her besties and she'll love you even more for scheduling it (who knows, you might even get lucky. wink, wink). And your daughter will grow up having a blast with her daddy and ultimately trying desperately to find a nice dude who's half the man you are.

WEEK 10: KEEPING FIT

Workout Routine; Baby Gym

For some, the descent into "Manland" is slow and gentle; for others it's steep and fast. It starts off innocently enough, as you spend the first couple of months absolutely fascinated with your new arrival. Nothing could be cuter or hold your attention more, and by week ten, your little girl is now showing more action than ever. Baby's arms are waving side to side, baby's legs are kicking up and down, and baby's butt is wiggling in every direction possible. But at this point, some of the newness has worn off and you might find yourself staring, laughing and being in complete awe a little less than the day before.

Instead, you might find yourself staring, laughing and being in complete disgust at the latest *Toddlers and Tiaras* episode on TLC *(The Learning Channel)*. This begins the inevitable return to the abyss us guys have come to know and love—a deep, immeasurable gulf known as Manland—the place where we sit on the couch wearing sweatpants, scratching ourselves, drinking beer and letting out a satisfying belch without a moment's notice. Of course, we all don't do that; moreover, we don't do that all the time, but we will start to find ourselves in this place more and more in-between the stages of "baby is new" and "infant is finally a toddler."

As idyllic as it sounds, spending time in Manland does have its consequences, most notably on your energy and activity levels. You may start to notice that it takes a second attempt to get off the couch. You'll have a long stretch once you're finally stable on your two legs. Your entire body will ache as you walk over to get another beverage from the fridge. I realize this may seem like a horrible image to most of you, but to a very small group of men, this becomes a disease that takes over and it's very difficult to treat. But as a new father, you need to know it's now or never. Are you going to embrace the challenges of maintaining a healthy, active lifestyle or are you going to take the easy road to an afternoon of Doritos, Miller Lite, and *SportsCenter?* Remember, your performance will impact you physically, your wife mentally, and your child developmentally. Last parting words of wisdom: pull yourself together and man up!

So, the Week 10 message is keep fit, and here are DADspirations to consider doing:

Establish a Workout Routine For Me

One early morning, our smoke detector started to chirp hellishly, and of course, never do the batteries run out at a decent hour. Whether I'm in the middle of winning the lottery or some other fantastically fantastic fantasy, smoke detector batteries always die between the hours of 2:00 a.m.to 5:00 a.m. I dragged myself out of bed, and as I passed by our full-length mirror in our bedroom I saw the image and thought, "Boy, that dude needs to work out." I didn't realize who that dude was until I had finished changing the batteries and found myself perspiring. I know what you're thinking, I can't possibly be that out of shape. Our condo surely must have been on fire, causing it to become so hot that I was sweating. Yes, that's much more realistic than the preposterous explanation that futzing with a smoke detector would result in such an intensive workout that I would have to dab my head with a towel after I finished. For argument's sake, let's just say that I might need to go to a gym. However, the arrival of Marie a couple of months ago all but guaranteed I wouldn't be spending 20 minutes to walk to the gym, 30 minutes on the treadmill, 30 minutes lifting weights, and walking another 20 minutes back home anymore. So what's a dad to do? Abandon Wifey and the kids for two hours a night so that I can watch fit 20-something's flirt with each other in tight clothes and know that will never be me again? As much as I feel that staying in shape and working out are important, I haven't reached the point where it's necessary for me to blow off my family.

Instead of going to the gym, I've brought the gym to me. Good-bye Bowflex PR3000, AudioStrider 990 Pro, and Incline Trainer X9i. Hello yoga mat, dumbbells, and my living room carpet. After the kiddies went to bed, I got back in shape, giving up the 40-minute travel time to do it. I spent three days a week at home, working out through army-inspired routines and dumbbell exercises, which first took just over an hour, but now take about 45 minutes. Put together a home workout routine that works best for you, whether it involves weights, a treadmill or milk cartons.

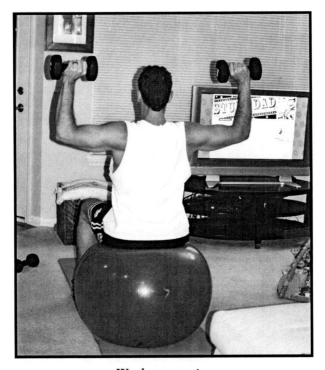

Workout routine

Baby Gym For My Daughter

No, I wasn't planning on taking Marie to Lifetime Fitness. But I did take her to the living room with me.

Since she couldn't stand up on her own yet, I couldn't imagine that encouraging sit-ups and push-ups would be a good use of my time or hers. The only exercise she had until then was tummy time on our bed, on the changing table, or on the hardwood floor. Since I turned the family room into my own gym, I thought it was only fair that Marie get her own gym too.

After researching the baby gym marketplace, I had to admit that her gym looked a lot more fun than mine. Most, if not all, gyms were themed (from rainforests to jungles to oceans), and equipped with music, bright lights, nature sounds, and lots of things to pull, push, and play with. Each had a soft, padded floor mat and silk-lined arches for attaching stuffed animals, mirrors or plastic rings. I looked back at my gray yoga mat and black dumbbells and sighed. Despite the giggling and cooing coming from Marie as she would playfully swat a toucan, I pressed on in my commitment to set a good example for my children. Plus it makes Marie the envy of other infants during her playdates, because even babies in diapers know who the cool kids with the fun toys are.

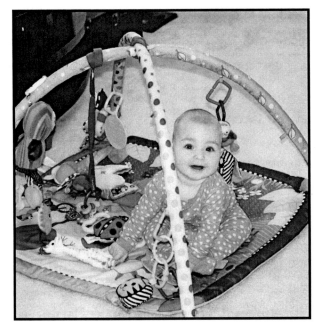

Baby gym

Baby Gym For a Son

Exercise is good for everyone; nothing needs to change based on girl or boy. Whether you have a son or daughter, any one of these gyms will do. If you want to go uber-boy, then pick out the jungle theme and watch him tangle with monkeys and wrestle crocodiles. These earn major man points at an early age, and bonus points if you get him to do a push-up, chin-up, sit-up or virtually any word with "up" attached to it. ('Throw-up' doesn't count, funny guy).

Week 10 Recap

The positive energy you have after working out is incredible. You feel happy for no reason, you begin to catch your wife surreptitiously checking out your butt, and you don't feel like going to sleep at 7:00 p.m. Yes, committing to the time is a challenge, but after a couple of weeks, you actually look forward to it. Sick, I know. And it's also good for baby. She gets sights, sounds and stimulation that will prepare her for the adrenaline rush of television, which we are trying to delay as long as possible.

WEEK 11: IT'S NEVER TOO EARLY TO PLAN

Top 10 Contest; College Fund

Blue eyes or brown? Blond hair or dark? Social butterfly or bookworm? These are the questions that Wifey and I debated during this week. However, like most parents, we were probably a little premature in talking about any of it, because Caucasian baby eyes don't change color until about six to nine months, if they are going to change at all. At eleven weeks, Marie was bald, and it would be another five months before we could actually start predicting. And she wasn't even remotely close to crawling, let alone talking or reading. So why do we ask ourselves these questions so early on in our little girl's life? Because we are parents, it's our job . . . and our compulsion.

While it's our job to plan ahead, see what's on the horizon, and be prepared, it's also just fun to sit around and talk about what she's going to be like when she grows up. Every time she giggled, I'd laugh and say, "She's going to be a comedian, just like Mommy!" Every time she cried, I'd sigh and say, "She's going to be fussy, just like Daddy." But every time she kicked her feet and swung her hands, Wifey and I both smiled proudly and said, "She's going to be athletic, just like both of us."

No matter what age Marie is, we are both going to be well ahead of her, getting ready for the ups and downs that are sure to come. But in the meantime, it can't hurt to anticipate what's to come. There are funny things to predict (Will she be a Kung Fu Master or Donut Tycoon?), and there are serious things to think about (disease, drugs, school). Find the balance that is right for your needs and wants for your child at the ages you feel is most appropriate.

So, the Week 11 message is it's never too early to plan. And here are DADspirations to consider doing:

Top 10 Contest For Me

For the most part, I like to keep things fun and light-hearted. I don't take myself too seriously and try my best to bring a sense of humor to any situation. And while I'm not a big gambler, I do like the excitement it can bring. Because Wifey and I had lots of guesses and proclamations about Marie's physical characteristics and personal development, it seemed only logical that these arguments would be best resolved by betting. So, we outlined ten milestones that some infants reach or don't reach by the end of year one, and we made our bets. When word got out to family and friends, they asked if they could get in on the action. I'm always open to some friendly competition, and thus an email went out to those closest to us. Below are the milestones that were measured:

1. Eye color (must be a solid color choice; blue-green or bluish-brown is just cheating).

2. Hair color (if she's still bald, this is a wash).

3. Number of teeth (must have fully come in, no turtles).

4. Whether she had a haircut (largely dependent on #2).

5. Will she be walking? (must be on her own, and no, standing and taking one step doesn't count)

6. Will she say both "mama" and "dada"? (must be said to the correct parent, not to Uncle Jimmy)

7. Will she be able to give a "high-5"? (must be done on command; if she swats at you because you're annoying her and it hits your hand by accident, it doesn't count).

8. Will Daddy have a classic "she pooped on me," "she peed on me," or "she did both on me" story?

9. Over/under five on the number of public places we will have abruptly left somewhere due to a Marie meltdown.

10. How far will she be able to throw Henry's Iowa Hawkeye Mini-Football? (this weighs about three pounds and we'll measure in inches, not yards).

11. Tie-breaker: What inappropriate word will Marie have mastered (e.g., profanity)? Parents have to promise no coaching of their specific word.

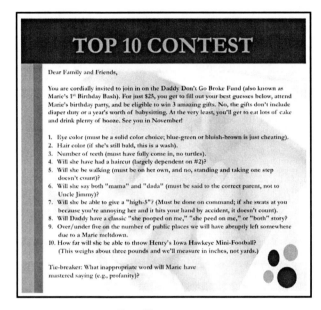

TOP 10 CONTEST

Dear Family and Friends,

You are cordially invited to join in on the Daddy Don't Go Broke Fund (also known as Marie's 1st Birthday Bash). For just $25, you get to fill out your best guesses below, attend Marie's birthday party, and be eligible to win 3 amazing gifts. No, the gifts don't include diaper duty or a year's worth of babysitting. At the very least, you'll get to eat lots of cake and drink plenty of booze. See you in November!

1. Eye color (must be a solid color choice; blue-green or bluish-brown is just cheating).
2. Hair color (if she's still bald, this is a wash).
3. Number of teeth (must have fully come in, no turtles).
4. Will she have had a haircut (largely dependent on #2)?
5. Will she be walking (must be on her own, and no, standing and taking one step doesn't count)?
6. Will she say both "mama" and "dada" (must be said to the correct parent, not to Uncle Jimmy)?
7. Will she be able to give a "high-5"? (Must be done on command; if she swats at you because you're annoying her and it hits your hand by accident, it doesn't count).
8. Will Daddy have a classic "she pooped on me," "she peed on me," or "both" story?
9. Over/under five on the number of public places we will have abruptly left somewhere due to a Marie meltdown.
10. How far will she be able to throw Henry's Iowa Hawkeye Mini-Football? (This weighs about three pounds and we'll measure in inches, not yards.)

Tie-breaker: What inappropriate word will Marie have mastered saying (e.g., profanity)?

Top Ten contest

You can also charge a $25 fee to enter the contest. What would the winners get? A weekend away with Marie? A year of paying her daycare fees? The right to buy Marie a couple of new boxes of diapers? No, this fee would get them a seat at Marie's 1-year birthday party, where the winners would be announced (1st, 1st runner-up, honorable mention). Not only will the prize money generate a lot of interest in keeping tabs on Marie, but it will also force them to come to the birthday party. And you know what that means? More people = more free stuff for Marie = less stuff Mommy and Daddy have to spend on Marie = more money we get to spend on ourselves = leather recliner? Projection TV? Bose surround-sound system? A father can dream, can't he?

College Fund for My Daughter

Would you miss $100 a paycheck? Me too. But I can stomach it, knowing I can set aside tax-free money for my daughter to go to college. At the rate of twice a month, twelve months a year, for eighteen years, we'll have a tidy nest egg for her. Now the good news is that it will amount to upwards of $40,000. The sobering news is that might only cover her freshman year. If you have a financial advisor, call him or her and it's a quick 30-minute meeting. If you don't, check out www.savingforcollege.com and look under 529 plans. You can review plans for each state and decide which plan is right for you. They offer a comprehensive, nationwide comparison and it's pretty easy to enroll. Twenty years ago, the average four-year university cost about $12,000 a year. Today, it costs approximately $20,000, which is nearly double. So looking

ahead to the year 2029 ... one year alone could amount to
~$40,000 a year??? Well, at least one year will be paid for.

College fund

College Fund for a Son

If you're convinced you have the next Michael Jordan
or Tiger Woods on your hands, guess again. Your kid
needs to go college. Spare me the "but he's an artist"

or "you don't need school to sing" routine. I know several people who didn't go to college for various reasons and, ten years later, are working the midnight shift at the local 7-11 (and no, they are not the owner of the establishment). Get your kid's ass in school, mortgage the next three lifetimes if you have to, but do it and make him or her earn that insanely expensive piece of paper that has a lot of fancy cursive writing on it.

Week 11 Recap

Yes, kids cost money, it's unavoidably true. But if you plan accordingly, like redistributing the funds provided by those closest to you in order to have a kick-ass home theater system or sacrificing a little bit of money now to find out that it wasn't nearly enough in the future, it might make you feel a little better about the cash your little ones will siphon over the next eighteen to twenty years.

WEEK 12: KEEP IT SIMPLE, KEEP IT FRESH

Life Lessons; Write a Story

She's almost three months old and already she has her own thoughts on life. Just last week, playing "Peek-A-Boo" would have my little girl giggling and smiling for nearly twenty minutes. Now that game seems to be yesterday's news, as she turns her head and looks away. I can tell she is done with it and ready for the next great Daddy-Daughter game.

I jogged my memory for the games we played with Henry and thought about stealing, er…, borrowing one for Marie. The two that came to mind were these:

- **"Jump Around":** I would hold Henry in my arms, crank up House of Pain's classic "Jump Around" and proceed to bounce around the house, eventually landing on a couch, bed or floor piled with pillows. Sure, it made me sweat like a pig and pissed off our condo neighbors, but Henry would giggle uncontrollably, which made it completely worth it.

- **"This Little Baby":** I would hold Henry in my arms as I recited a revised version of the famous poem, as we hurried from one room to the next. *This little baby went to kitchen, this little baby stayed in bed. This little baby liked the great room, this little baby preferred the den. And this little baby went.... "waa waa waa" all the way back to bed.* And we'd flop onto the bed and giggle for the next ten minutes.

There were a few more songs that were "Henry-ified" that made for some personalized interaction that brings out parents' personalities. Apparently, we are adrenaline-crazed parents who make their kid laugh by running around the house and crash-landing on various pieces of furniture.

We didn't reinvent the wheel; we kept things simple and fun. And with Marie, we knew that we'd have to change things up with her as she's a completely different animal (sorry honey) from her brother. Ripping off what we did with Henry didn't feel right, because it didn't feel like Marie. It felt like dressing her in Henry's collared onesie and plaid shorts. She needed something fresh, something personal to her.

So, the Week 12 message is keep it simple, keep it fresh. And here are DADspirations to consider doing:

Life Lessons For Me

I have a short memory, as my wife will vouch. She will say something important; I'll forget about it a week later. I'll say something funny, and I'll forget about it a day later. And when I think of something really inspiring and thoughtful, I usually forget it about an hour later. I forget all of these things, unless I write them down—if I have a pen and paper handy. Thankfully, my smartphone is glued to my hip, which has a NOTES application. With a simple touch of the NOTES icon, the application opens up so I can type my thoughts whenever, wherever. For me, I need to capture these nuggets of wisdom immediately, because I have trouble remembering what day it is, let alone trying to recall a thought I had on the train, at 6:00 a.m., after four hours of sleep, while trying to memorize my presentation to senior management at 8:00 a.m.

Here are five of my favorite nuggets:

- You are beautiful, every hour of every day, and you don't need to be a stick figure or wear make-up to prove it.

- Being mean and bitchy is wasteful energy; life is much more fun when you are smiling, laughing and being nice to people.

- Go for it, always. Life's too short for regrets and the 'woulda coulda shouldas.' Don't go through life without trying everything at least once. Whoa, wait a second—there are several things you should definitely NOT try, but I will wait until you are sixteen for that discussion.

- Trust is earned and not to be assumed. What you say or type is going to be repeated and tweeted to your best friend's cousin's step-sister's neighbor's boyfriend who lives in Europe, in under ten minutes.

- You are not entitled to anything. You want to play sports? Practice. You want a scholarship? Study. You want to make a million bucks? You will need to work… hard.

Notes **Life Lessons** +

Life Lessons
1. You are beautiful, every hour of every day.
2. Being mean and bitchy is wasteful energy.
3. Go for it, always.
4. Trust is earned and not be assumed.
5. No one owes you anything.
6. You can tell me anything, anytime.
7. I'm always here for you when you

Life lessons

Writing a Story For My Daughter

I know she won't be able read it today, tomorrow, or the next day, but someday she will; and until then, she'll just have to listen to me read it. Whether it's a Saturday afternoon or before bedtime, she'll likely know this story by heart before she's even able to read it. But it's something I made just for her, something to let her know that Daddy thinks she is pretty darn special. We know everyone loves pictures, including 3-month olds. So, using Microsoft PowerPoint, I collected old photos from a trip to Toronto that Wifey and I took a couple years back, and told my story over 20 slides. Using Power-Point allows me flexibility to read off a print-out or, if I'm in a pinch, open it and view it from my smartphone. It includes a princess, a good guy dressed in white, a bad guy wearing black, a wacky side-kick, and an improbable, harrowing journey—oh, you heard this one before?

Well, here's the kicker. The message is not like one you've heard before. My daughter won't learn to treat others how she wishes to be treated, or that every action has a consequence, or always to pursue one's dreams. No, no, no, I'll leave that to the fine folks at Disney.

While my story's structure will be familiar, the message will not. It's a unique, but clear message that needs to be instilled in the majority of girls in this country, and it's simple to understand, even simpler to follow. The main message of this story is don't date until you've gotten you're first full-time job. Yes, I know that sounds like I'm an overbearing, uber-protective father. And you know what? I probably am and I'm okay with it. What I've learned in my 30-plus years of life is that kids will always do things earlier than you tell them to:

- 'No smoking until you're 18' means that kids will try it freshman year of high school.

- 'No alcohol until you're 21' means that kids will be drinking their junior year of high school.

- 'No boyfriends until they've been enrolled into a 401k' means my kid will go on her first date in college, when she's not living at home, when I can't get in the car and follow them, and when I will not really know anything about it. Mission accomplished.

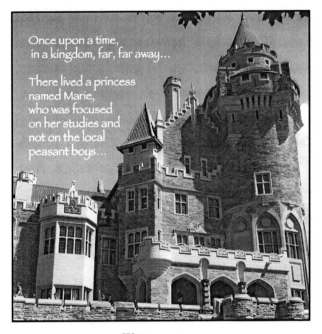

Write a story

Writing a Story For a Son

You miss every shot you don't take? Very insightful, Wayne Gretzky. Leaders aren't born, they are made? Incredibly inspiring, Vince Lombardi. I've failed over and over and over again in my life. And that is why I succeed? Not bad, Michael Jordan. Eh, those stories are all overplayed. This story needs an original theme, one that transcends sports—a story about ensuring one's own future. Yes, I've got it. This story should be about "wrapping it up." I admit, it's simplistic and crude, but when your son is disease-free and childfree on his wedding day, then 'Congratulations Dad!' You get the biggest gold star that was ever made.

Week 12 Recap

I want to be the best dad possible, looking out for my little girl even when she's not such a little girl anymore. The world will constantly change, and I'm guessing not for the better. The biggest worry I had in high school was how to get alcohol. Kids now have to worry if some kid who is disgruntled is going to shoot up the school one day. All I want to do is remind her of all of things she needs to know to make that world a little easier, safer and as enjoyable as possible.

MONTH 4

WEEK 13: RELAX, YOU'VE EARNED IT

Boys' Night Out; Favorite Movie

You are heading into baby's three-month birthday. I don't know about you, but it's been an exhausting process for me and for Wifey too. Sorry, honey. Marie's middle-of-the-night feedings, her wailing for no rhyme or reason, the constant attention she demands, while we're trying to train, teach and track down Henry, has left Wifey and me beat. But don't let the little girl wear you down; you only have eighteen more years of this before you turn her loose! You're right, loose is probably not the best word to associate with your daughter.

It's important to remember that you do have a life outside the home—and at the right time, in the right place, it's healthy to remember that life. Those buddies you used to talk and text to just a few months ago? They are still there; don't forget about them. They will be your sounding board, the people you vent to; and whether they have kids or not, they won't judge you. Hell, they will probably ignore what you say and they probably won't answer you, but that's not what you need, is it? You need a break. You need to spend a few hours being the guy you used to be. This won't be a nightly, or even weekly, occurrence and you probably don't want it to be (hopefully). Just take a few hours to do whatever it was that you used to do on a Friday night. Video games, bars, sporting events; call your buddies, make plans, and don't, even for a second, feel guilty about it. Wifey and baby will be fine without you for a few hours, and you know what? You'll start to miss them, look forward to seeing them and walk in your front door later that night happier to be home than you ever have before (and if you want another BNO, it better not be in the morning).

By the end of this week (at the time of this writing), there will be just nine days left until my daughter's first 100 days, and for that final week, I'll be doing something every day for her. That is why I need to rest up, chill out and get ready for the final push.

So, the Week 13 message is relax—you've earned it; and here are DADspirations to consider doing:

Boys Night Out For Me

I'm not asking for Bulls courtside seats or a Blackhawks game at center ice, just a few hours at a bar with my close buddies, known as The Four Horsemen. I might be watching a random basketball game, betting on the next team to hit a three, eating a plate full of cheese fries before my basket of hot wings comes out, and drinking whatever beer special they have on tap, even if it comes with a magic bullet. I don't want to take part of any conversation that doesn't have us arguing over the reasons for the Blackhawks' sudden collapse, debating whether the Bulls need Dwight Howard, or examining what the White Sox's chances are for winning the AL Central. Any other topic comes up, and

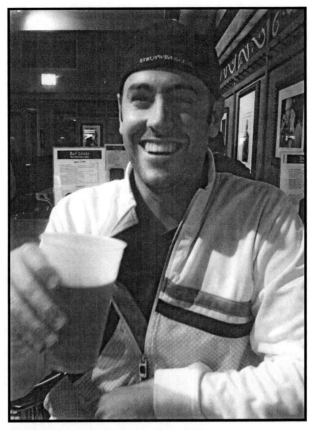

Boys' night out

I'm going to shut up. I don't care about a half-naked Rob Gronkowski partying with strippers after the Super Bowl loss (the NFL season is over). I don't care about how Kentucky's freshmen make them the best team in college (it's not March yet, so college basketball is meaningless right now). And I don't care about Urban Meyer being an asshole and poaching recruits (real football is only played on Sundays). I want to talk Bulls, Hawks and Sox. And if anyone wants to talk about family, wives or kids, I'm going to pour their beer over their head.

Show Favorite Movie For My Daughter

One is never too young to be introduced to the Western movie genre, even at three months of age. This particular weekend, Marie and I are going to plop onto the couch and we are going to watch Tombstone—two hours of men being men, in a more primitive time when men rode horses, wore brimmed hats, and felt free to be trigger happy. If someone was being rude, you'd shoot 'em. If someone was acting stupid, you'd shoot 'em. If someone pissed you off, you'd shoot 'em.

Will Marie understand this? Of course not, but maybe in the years to come, she will. This is because I'm going to watch this movie every year with her until she leaves for college so she knows this movie inside and out. This movie will toughen her up for the cruel world that awaits her. And when she finds herself in an uncomfortable situation with a boy at school, when Daddy is not around to protect her, she can pull strength and courage from this movie. Marie will stand tall, remain cool, and confidently quote the classic Doc Holliday line from Tombstone, "I'll be your Huckleberry," which will surely drive chills down said boy's spine.

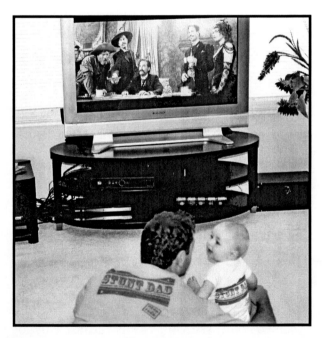

Favorite movie

Show Favorite Movie for a Son

No need to change anything here. Just know that when your son is old enough to understand what's going on in the movie (age three or four), you'd better be prepared for him to walk around recreating movie scenes for at least a month after viewing the movie. For me, when I'm about to reprimand Marie at the age of five, and she responds with squinty eyes, leans right into my face and mutters my favorite line from Tombstone, *"Listen here Mr. Law Dog, law don't go around here. Savvy?"* I'm pretty sure it will feel like the proudest moment of my life.

Week 13 Recap

Preparing for the final days of a 100-day challenge requires two things: commitment and downtime. And after thirteen weeks, you've earned some downtime. Call up your buddies and grab some beer, or grab your little boy or girl, snuggle them into the couch, and enjoy a great movie. Either way, you are relaxing, rejuvenating and getting ready to take on that final week.

NINE DAYS OF DOTING

DAY 92: PAINT THE TOWN RED

Daddy and Daughter Date

Until now, baby has left the house only out of necessity, as we didn't want to expose her to unwanted germs. But don't be afraid: the outdoors is a good thing. She sees new sights, smells new smells, and hears new sounds. And you get to remember what fresh air feels like, away from a house that needs to be cleaned, away from the dirty clothes that seem never to stop piling up and away from your wife who always has something to say.

So, the Day 92 message is paint the town red. And here is a DADspiration to consider doing:

Take Daughter Out on a Date

It was our first date. I was a little nervous, a little anxious, and a little frustrated. The last first date I had been on, I ended up marrying the girl, so I felt a little pressure with Marie. However, I did make the list below to help keep me cool, calm and collected and remind me of the key first date dos and don'ts with my baby girl.

- **Keep it nice and easy:** Don't feel compelled to spend hundreds of dollars trying to impress her; she's only three months old: her expectations will never be lower.

- **Be early and bring flowers:** Show her this is important to you and that she's not just another baby you're taking out.

- **Age is just a number:** Don't get hung up on the 33-year age difference; it's your daughter; she will love you despite not understanding your John Hughes references.

- **Avoid other eye candy:** Don't go to parks or malls where your daughter will feel the need to compete with other babies for your attention; keep the date private and all about her.

- **Dress to impress:** It's your daughter, not a doll, which means she has feelings too and wants to be with someone presentable in public too; no scruff, no sweats and no sandals.

- **Don't forget protection:** She will surprise you at the worst moment—probably twice—so remember to bring extra diapes and wipes, at least two bottles of milk, and three different outfits for her.

- **Do your homework:** She doesn't have a Facebook or LinkedIn page you can stalk, but she does have a mom. Suck it up and ask Wifey for a few tips and tricks, because she knows her so, so much better than you could ever imagine.

- **Don't drink and date:** Just one beer? It means you are in a bar. Which means you are a horrible father. It's your first date with your daughter and you can't go three hours without a drink? You should be fired, immediately.

- **Stay positive:** You might get thrown up on, she might have a wicked blowout and she might start wailing for no reason. This does not wipe the smile off your face. This does not make you think about heading home early. This does not let you be anything less than the cheery, excited, rockstar of a dad that you are.

- **Eat what you want:** Just because she decides on "just milk," don't let that stop you from getting a hamburger, hot wings or pizza. Having "just a salad" won't impress her.

- **Act interested in her:** Don't spend the entire time playing "Words With Friends," talking on your cell phone or gazing off into the distance. Ask her questions, maintain eye contact, laugh when she laughs.

- **This is not your personal therapy session:** Do not bitch about your job, complain about the bills you pay, or lecture her about boys. Talk to her, find out what makes her smile, coo and giggle.

- **Don't over-analyze her:** If she stares off into the distance, it doesn't mean you're boring—she is probably just mesmerized by the life we take for granted. After all, she is fresh out of her own version of solitary confinement, so even the tweet of a bird is likely to set off an explosion of senses throughout her body. If she frowns from time to time, it doesn't mean she doesn't like you—she is probably just trying to poop. And if one minute she smiles, the next minute she cries, it doesn't mean you don't understand her—she is probably trying to decide if she wants to sleep or stay awake.

- **Don't talk about her older siblings:** Keep your other children out of this. Don't talk about how the older brother is such a great athlete or the older sister will become a movie star someday; it'll come across as favoritism and create a feeling of bitterness.

- **Be yourself:** If you're funny, tell her jokes. If you're romantic, tell her about the sweet things you've done for your wife. If you're boring, tell her about the weather. Just don't be someone you're not; behind those eyes is a soul who will see right through you.

- **Give compliments:** Just because she can't tell you how hot and sexy you are doesn't mean she doesn't want to be, or deserve to be called beautiful, cute, adorable, sweet, angelic, loveable, the one and only, the light of your life…. Remember, this is not about you.

- **Kill 'er with kindness:** Over and over and over, tell her three words. As often as you can, say I LOVE YOU. True, it's just a first date and this is a pretty over-the-top feeling, but when you feel it, you feel it—right?

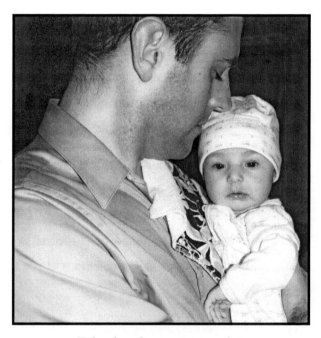

Take daughter out on a date

Take a Son Out on a Date

Okay, the idea is spot on, but the approach will need to change. You're not taking your son 'on a date.' You'll take him somewhere to 'hang out.' But just because it's boys' day out doesn't mean you should take him to a bar. It's not boys' night out. Your new version of Sunday Funday should involve parks, courts, or pools, not shots, darts, or stools. Consider taking the little guy to an empty baseball field, let him play on the grass, and show him what it means to be a man.

DAY 93: BUILD IT AND SHE WILL COME: TOY BOX

One week left and I've just realized that I've been too soft with my daughter. From the songwriting, to the dance lessons, to the monthly photos, most of the things I've done for Marie have been—well, girly.

I don't want her to be thinking that daddy is anything less than a Tim 'The Toolman' Taylor from *Home Improvement,* so it's time to get my hands dirty, time to show her why men were born to wield power tools, time to show her why men are men. I know what you're thinking: *"He's going to hop in that damn tractor of his and build his daughter a damn baseball diamond in the middle of his cornfield. This guy is cracking, just seven days short of his goal!"* Sorry to disappoint you, this is not *Field of Dreams;* I'm not hearing voices and my name is not Ray Kinsella.

But the Day 93 message *is* build it and she will come, and here is a DADspiration to consider doing:

Building a Toy Box For My Daughter

I'm not grabbing five pieces of wood, hammering nails into each of the corners, and painting her name on the box. That's bush league. If my daughter is going to get an education in Building Stuff 101, then this toy box is going to kick ass. After searching the Internet for some plans, I came across a Chalk Box: a multi-purpose box that is "toy storage meets chalkboard." However, chalk to me sounds like a pain in the ass to clean up, so I am replacing the chalkboard element with a dry erase board. How badass is this? Not only will Marie get to chuck all her toys in the box, she can get her creative juices flowing from the time she's one up through grammar school. After convincing Wifey to take the kids elsewhere for the afternoon, I got to spend the afternoon in the garage cutting plywood, hammering nails and drinking Miller Lite. I'm considering this a major win-win for the both of us.

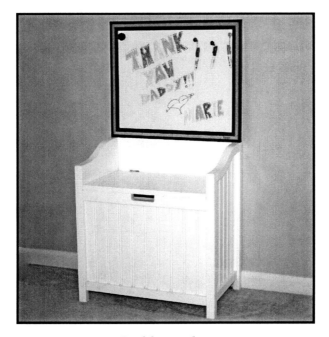

Build a toy box

Building a Toy Box For a Son

Power tools, building stuff, and markers? This idea is way too cool not to share it with either a boy or a girl. The first thing written on the dry erase board should read, "Dad is a stud. Love, your little buddy." And if you are feeling especially dude-ish, we all know men love fire at any age, as noted in Week 7. Find some stickers depicting flames, slap 'em all over the box, and you've earned your major 'street cred' with neighboring dads.

DAY 94: SOMEONE LIKE YOU: ALMA MATER GEAR

Under a week to go and we've watched our little girl grow like a weed. She has completely outgrown the 0-3 outfits and most of her 3-6s. She fits comfortably into clothes that she shouldn't be in for another three months, which makes me think that she'll need eighteen-month clothes when she turns one.

This is great news, because it means she will likely be walking this November, which is THE time of year for college sports. College football is winding down and college basketball is heating up. And what better way to celebrate this time than by showing off where Mommy and Daddy went to college. Fortunately for Marie, we both have the same alma mater: The University of Iowa, home of the Hawkeyes. Unfortunately for Marie, I am a sucker for matching outfits for parents and baby. Some people love this; some people are nauseated by it. You can see where this is going: I 'heart' coordination.

So, the Day 94 message is "Someone like you" (luckily Marie is too young to object). And here is a DADspiration to consider doing:

Alma Mater Gear For My Daughter

Since Marie, is going to need to be ready for tailgating, I'm going to start loading up on our alma mater football gear for her AND me. This will include the following plethora of Iowa Hawkeyes gear:

- **Football jerseys:** Any self-respecting fan wears this to a football game, so we might as well have her start from day one.

- **Sippy cup:** Whether it's milk or water, she's got to have something to chug it down with.

- **Camo beanie cap:** It's Iowa, and sadly, this is actually a fashion statement.

- **Booties:** Again, it's Iowa—a warm day in November is slightly above freezing.

- **Chuck Taylors:** The girl will need some kind of style to combat the Camo.

- **Jammies:** After a hard day of partying and cheering, she'll need something to pass out in.

Tailgate Gear For a Son

You will be tempted to purchase a beer holder hat and have your son walking around the tailgate sucking Miller Lite through a transparent, flexible straw. Should this happen before his first birthday, you are destined to raise him to be a raging alcoholic before he gets his driver's license. My advice? Stick to tradition with a jersey, a hat and pajamas.

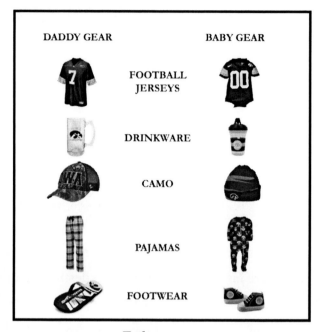

DADDY GEAR   BABY GEAR

FOOTBALL
JERSEYS

DRINKWARE

CAMO

PAJAMAS

FOOTWEAR

Tailgate gear

DAY 95: THE BEST IDEAS ARE ALWAYS BORROWED

Black and White Photos

Since Marie is our second child, Wifey and I know recycling all too well. Even though our first child was a boy, we were able to re-use a lot of the same clothes, equipment and necessities for Marie.

One of the more valuable things I've learned as a parent is thriftiness, which is a nice word for being cheap. Money seems to go out quicker than it comes in, so I am always looking to save a buck, re-purpose things or generally spend less whenever I can. So building off that idea, I thought back to Week 2's message of *Bond Before It's Too Late* and am re-using some of the photos from our professional photo shoot.

So, the Day 95 message is the best ideas are always borrowed. And here is a DADspiration to consider doing:

Black and White Canvas Photos of My Daughter

Our one-hour photo shoot in Week 2 resulted in over 200 photos. About ten of them have been put into frames around our house and offices; the rest were posted to Facebook. Other than that, they appear on our Apple TV whenever we listen to music and look at photos, which has happened exactly twice since she was born. Needless to say, we haven't gotten the full value of the money that we spent on the photo shoot. That is, until now.

I selected three of those pictures, a close-up of her profile (because she has the cutest little chubby cheeks known to mankind), a hand (because her fingers are so long and dainty, like her English grandmother) and a foot (because they were just downright gigantic like her Sasquatch of a father). Through an online store called Gafy.com, I had those pictures printed out in black and white at 8" x 8" on canvas and stretched and mounted on a wood frame. It's simple, it's artistic and we have a great spot to show-case them on the stairway wall leading into her bedroom.

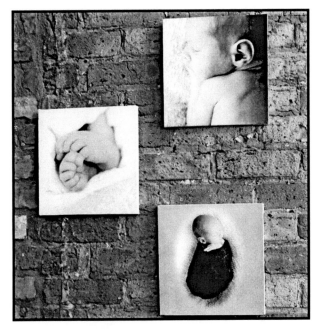

Black and white photos

Black and White Canvas Photos of a Son

Since you aren't focused on showcasing the obvious differences between baby girls and boys, at least I hope to God you aren't, then nothing needs to change for a son. The same adorable little ears, nose or lips on a girl are just as adorable on a boy.

DAY 96: REKINDLE THE FIRE: GRANDPARENTS' DAY

With just four days left until 100 days, I had an epiphany. It's funny how great ideas always seem to come at the last minute, after you spent so much time thinking, planning and doing. You get to the end of a project, and BOOM, the light shines down upon you.

For this stroke of genius, since Wifey's parents live in Canada, they were out of the question. However, even though my parents live nearby, I have not taken advantage of that nearly as much as I should. So, as the wonderful son and loving father that I am, I only have my parents' best interests at heart with this idea. In order to bring them closer to their grandchild, now would be an excellent time to implement this idea. The genius idea? Have a Grandparents' Day! And it just so happens that it also would give Wifey and me some much needed one-to-one time. Or if I play my cards right, it will be "one-*on*-one" time. Wink, wink.

So, the Day 96 message is rekindle the fire. And here is a DADspiration to consider doing:

Grandparents' Day with My Daughter

Yes, I realize that there is a Hallmark Holiday established for this, but this is a different kind of Grandparents' Day. This day won't actually be celebrating Grandma and Grandpa (sorry, Mom and Dad). This day will be celebrating a day away from Marie. Sounds horrible, doesn't it? I mean, who would want to spend the day away from their beautiful, adorable, baby girl? She's only this age once in her life; you should never want to be away from her. But for argument's sake, let's imagine, just for one second—what a couple could do with this time to themselves.

- Walk downtown and grab coffee and breakfast at an old-school diner.

- Walk back home and sleep until noon.

- Eat grilled cheese sandwiches and Doritos for lunch while you sit in your Snuggie on the couch and watch an uninterrupted movie...in the daytime.

- Read a book, an actual book that doesn't contain cartoon animals, three sentences on a page, or rhymes.

- Cook a dinner that doesn't involve a microwave and actually be able to eat a warm meal together for the first time in three months.

- Go to sleep at 10:00 p.m. and not be woken up until 10:00 a.m. the following morning.

Oh, the list is endless. I could fill a novel with the things we could do. But wait—how could we pawn off our kid on my parents? Yes, this is a horrible idea. How could we even think about doing such a thing? It's so very, very selfish on our part, almost like we want to have some fun like it's 2009 B.K. (Before Kids). What kind of parents are we? Sane ones.

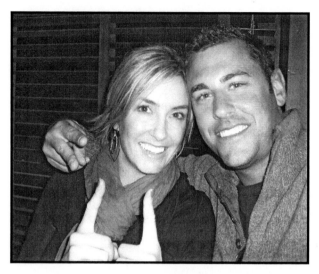

Grandparents' Day

Grandparents' Day for a Son

This is another non-gender biased idea that works just as well with your little prince as it would for a princess. After all, this is really about you anyway, so who really cares whether it's geared toward a girl or boy? As long as the kid is breathing, has no visible scarring and hasn't lost a significant amount of blood by the time you pick him up the next day, consider the day a major success.

DAY 97: KEEP YOUR FAMILY CLOSE AND YOUR RELATIVES CLOSER

Family Photo Poster

In a perfect world, my kids would see much, much more of our family than they currently do. One set of relatives lives in Canada, another group lives in California, and we live in Chicago. Aside from my parents and my brother's family, the majority of our family members do not live close by.

Since, in our household, we hold family in high regard, I want our little ones to know our relatives, whether they see them every other year or every ten years. I want our children to recognize an uncle when he walks in the door or get excited to see their cousin whom they haven't seen in a year. So instead of relying on sporadic visits to or from family, I'm going to bring family to us. While I'm not thinking about taking on permanent live-ins or building life-size, cardboard cut-outs of everyone, I do like the idea of keeping their images in constant view of Marie.

So, the Day 97 message is to keep your family close and your relatives closer. And here is a DADspiration to consider doing:

Family Photo Poster For My Daughter

I took pictures of 26 family members (fortunately, I have a big family) and made a poster of them. This isn't, however, your typical family collage. Since Marie is only three months old, based upon our experience with her older brother at that age, she is probably going to respond more to cartoons than to real-life images. Using those 26 pictures, I created photo caricatures of them, using a free service from a cartoon photo website. Each cartoon replication of a relative was assigned a letter of the alphabet. It got a little tricky with some of the lesser used letters of the alphabet, so I couldn't always assign the first letter of the name (e.g., Alex, Elizabeth) and a couple I had to completely make up, but it's for the good of the kid, right? Qim instead of Kim? Yep, I'll have to explain that one in a few years. Additionally, Marie's room is themed with chocolate brown, green and pink colors so those were used as the basis for the poster—and no, poopy diapers weren't the inspiration for this. The final poster measured 11" x 17" and the only costs came from a $9.99 white frame from Target. Is it Picasso? No. Is it perfect? Absolutely. It's the first thing Marie sees in the morning when we walk through each of the pictures and names, and the last thing she sees before bed time.

Family Photo Poster For a Son

Brown, green and pink aren't the most masculine of colors, but hey, if you're into that, and into permanently damaging your son for life, go for it! I'm going to just assume relatives would stay the same if you had a girl or boy, but if you prefer something dark and twisted that would alter your family tree, best to keep that to yourself.

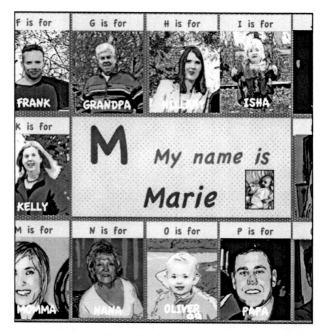

Family photo poster

DAY 98: THE WORLD IS WAITING

Plane Ticket

One of the best experiences of my life occurred three months after I graduated from college. I boarded a plane, flew halfway around the world to Melbourne, Australia and backpacked up and down the eastern coastline for twelve months. I saw a part of the world that most people only read about in magazines. I met people from more countries than I can remember. And I left Australia a completely different person than when I entered.

Do I think it should be a law that young adults spend time outside of our country, meeting people from around the world, and experiencing different cultures? Absolutely. I think it should be written in stone that life is too short to spend it in the state of Illinois or whatever the state or province in which one grows up. The United States totals 3,794,083 square miles, accounting for just 2% of the Earth's total surface. My country is a blip on a map. How does yours stack up? Thought so. So do yourself and your children a favor and get them the hell out of your motherland to experience another part of this Earth.

So, the Day 98 message is the world is waiting. And here is a DADspiration to consider doing:

Plane Ticket Out of the Country For My Daughter

No, I'm not sending my three-month-old daughter to Australia. But for the next 22 years, I will be putting away $10 a month for my daughter to use toward a plane ticket out of the U.S. when she graduates from college. And yes, she will be graduating from college. Will $2,500+ cover her plane ticket twenty years from now? Not sure, but it should help. One of the biggest barriers to leaving our country is the money it costs to go somewhere else, whether it's Mom and Dad wondering how to shell out another two grand for tickets or a young adult wondering how many burgers he or she will need to flip at McDonald's. But thanks to banking's automated transfer service, I can set this up tomorrow, completely forget about it, and space out for the next couple of decades. On her graduation day, when other kids are going to be getting career advice, framed diplomas or a stuffed teddy bear in a graduation gown, Marie will receive a plane ticket to the destination of her choice. Where she goes and how soon she returns is something I can't predict, but I will guarantee one thing—she will have the time of her life, just like her daddy did.

Plane Ticket Out of the Country For a Son

Truth be told, I'm a lot more comfortable with this idea for my son. A daughter roaming the foothills of Europe or a son trekking his way up and down mountaintops? I'd prefer the latter. However, after daddy's strong urging, when Marie achieves her black belt in martial arts, completes four years of combat training and graduates with honors in beating the crap out of would-be attackers, then I will sleep better at night while she's checking out the best beaches Thailand has to offer.

Additionally, having just watched the movie *Taken*, I can admit that I am more of a Larry David than a Liam

Neeson. All the more reason Marie needs to become her own secret spy.

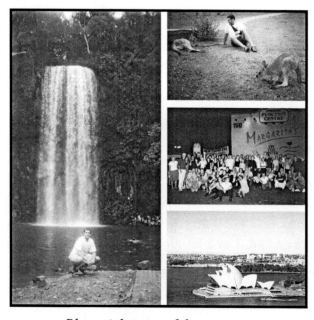

Plane ticket out of the country

DAY 99: PRIDE, DON'T HIDE

Baby Print Artwork

I didn't realize how much Marie had grown until we took her monthly photos this week. Gone was her sleepy-eyed expression. Gone was the fist-clenching and toe-curling. Gone was the little bundle of wrinkles. Here is this bright-eyed, long and lean little girl. She definitely has her mommy's looks and physical traits, which is a very good thing, because me with long hair is not a good look. But my narcissistic side immediately noticed the two characteristics she'd picked up from Daddy: big hands and even bigger feet.

Now, I could worry that she will grow up to be Amazonian or a female Sasquatch, but that's not what's keeping me up at night. Rather, I'm concerned she's going to be taller than her older brother. Nothing gives a boy a Napoleon complex more than being shorter than a girl, especially when she lives in the room right next to his. The thought of hearing screams from the two of them fighting and knowing those shrieks could be coming from Henry is enough to make Dad wake up in a cold sweat at 3:00 a.m.

All kidding aside, I'm going to do the exact opposite and show off her hands and feet. However, instead of traumatizing Marie for life by putting these features on a pedestal for all to see, I have a plan to artistically showcase these features so people *aww* instead of *eww*. Using a rainbow of colors and incorporating cute animals will turn these hands and feet into the most adorable body parts one has ever seen.

So, the Day 99 message is pride, don't hide. And here is a DADspiration to consider doing:

Baby Print Artwork For My Daughter

I love the idea of creatively capturing Marie's hand and feet prints, and a unique way to do that is to make canvas posters of them. While this is similar to the black and white canvas photos I made, there is something extra special about artistically capturing them as well. Whether it's the color, the unique shapes or just the simplicity of it, they will bring a great splash of color and freshness. Here's how to do it: Grab some paint, grab those feet, dip 'em, and stick 'em onto a piece of white canvas. After the paint dries (you've of course removed your child from said canvas), use a marker to draw the design of a butterfly in-between each of the footprints. Do that three times on each separate piece of canvas; hang them in her bedroom; and call it a day. Who knew you had such creativity inside of you? Definitely not your wife. Put these babies up on the wall, and watch your wife melt over how sweet and thoughtful you are. In advance, you're welcome.

Baby Print Artwork For a Son

Butterfly? Sure, that's cute, that will work. Or, let's say you have a son whose hands rival those of an orangutan. You could dip those mitts into paint, stick 'em onto the white canvas, darken the fingertips, and draw a set of eyes in the thumb area, with antlers just above each thumb. Now you're looking at a strong, manly moose. Or if the winter holidays are soon approaching, redden one of the noses, and presto! You now have Rudolph and his reindeer. Either way, slap the piece into a nice (cheap) frame and you are golden!

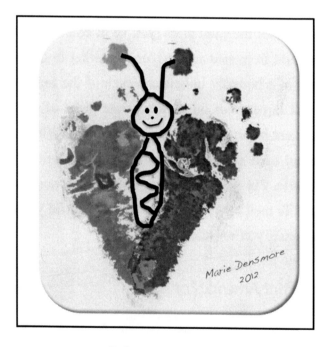

Baby print artwork

DAY 100: PROOF IS IN THE CAMCORDER

Video Record

I don't know what's more difficult to believe: that this project is coming to an end or that my daughter is almost four months old. Time has certainly flown by, and while I've done some great things to remember this special time, such as her Time Capsule and Monthly Photo Journal, I haven't really been able to capture her movements or her sounds. This is the stage in life where she is full of giggles, smiles and coos—just because she can.

This is also a stage that she will never remember, no matter how you try to explain it to her when she's older. When she's five, she'll be able to remember what life was like at age three. But when she's three, she won't be able to remember a thing. So, as much as this is captured for Wifey and me, it's also to prove to Marie visually that she really was this tiny. And when she is throwing a tantrum, it would be nice to play the video and remind her that she was actually a sweet little happy bunny of a girl once upon a time.

So, the Day 100 message is proof is in the camcorder. And here is a DADspiration to consider doing:

Video Record My Daughter

God, video recording my daughter sounds inappropriate, doesn't it? Or do I just have a jaded mind? Well maybe a little, but the real idea here is to get a good quality recording. This means not using an iPhone™ video, which ends up completely sucking when you try watching it on anything other than your two-inch phone screen. Buy, rent or borrow a real video recorder to get a good quality recording, one with high enough resolution for a plasma screen and that can withstand the test of time. After all, these kinds of things are pulled out for weddings and baby showers, right? Or dare I attempt replicating the famous Google commercial and email the video to a personal email address that I set up for her, also preparing the way for hundreds of other future email messages. It's not an original idea, but it's still pretty damn cute. Either way, I need Marie's hands wiggling and mouth giggling at 1080p resolution, the highest of the high definition. For the last thing I do in the first 100 days, I want it to be something that will show her off now and twenty years from now, something that is timeless, something that will last forever. And with this video I couldn't think of a better way to wrap up her first 100 days.

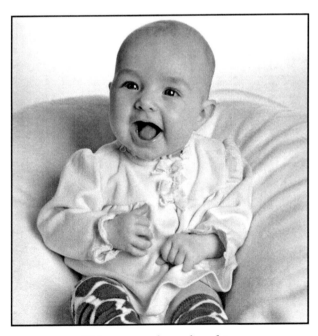

Video record my daughter

Video Record a Son

It doesn't sound nearly as bad, but the same general approach applies here. Keep in mind, whether the video is for a boy or girl, I highly recommend keeping your video star fully clothed. As much as you might think he has the world's most adorable tummy or butt, you run the risk of "accidental capture." Meaning, when this video gets replayed at a wedding reception, the last thing everyone, especially the groom, wants to see is his little willy. Trust me, you will have done your due diligence as a father by embarrassing him more than enough up until that point, Dad.

IN CONCLUSION

No, you didn't solve your family's economic crisis like FDR helped solve the United States crisis in the 1930s. But we all know that no amount of programs would ever be enough to get us, as a family, out of the debt and mounting bills that pile up week after week.

However, you did what most other Dads didn't, couldn't, or wouldn't. You've spent the past 100 days thinking about those who matter most to you, more than anyone expected of you. You exceeded all expectations. Your family is in awe, your wife is astonished, and your little girl (or boy) is so appreciative, whether she or he realizes it.

This was more than just getting through 100 days of "doing stuff" for you and your kid. This was bigger than that, much bigger. By demonstrating fun, proactive ways to bring joy, passion and love into your family, you've established an attitude and tone for how much of a rock-star dad you are going to be to your family for the next twenty years.

FDR had his "3 Rs": *Relief, Recovery,* and *Reform. Relief* for the unemployed and poor; *Recovery* of the economy to normal levels; and *Reform* of the financial system to prevent a repeat Depression.

You now have your own "3 Rs": *Regard, Remember,* and *Relish. Regard* your wife with the same importance as you do yourself. *Remember* you still need to have time set aside for yourself. And *relish* your angelic, adorable, and amazing little newborn every second of every day.

ABOUT THE AUTHOR

Father of two, Pete Densmore doesn't consider himself an expert in parenthood by any means. He makes the same number of mistakes as every other parent and doesn't have any fancy combination of letters after his name. However, the author has given much thought about and learned through experience what makes a father an inspired parent. Equally important, he presents ideas that new fathers can use to keep themselves and their wives happy, and to help keep their marriages from suffering under the strain and demands of child-rearing. Densmore believes that anyone can be an inspired dad as long as he wants to put the time, effort and heart into becoming one.

CPSIA information can be obtained at www.ICGtesting.com
Printed in the USA
BVOW03s0211031213

338003BV00007B/61/P